T0255839

THE LITTLE BOOK of PEDIATRICS

Infants to Teens and
Everything In Between

THE LITTLE BOOK of PEDIATRICS

Infants to Teens and Everything In Between

MICHAEL J. STEINER, MD, MPH
UNC SCHOOL OF MEDICINE
DEPARTMENT OF PEDIATRICS
CHAPEL HILL, NORTH CAROLINA

KELLY S. KIMPLE, MD, MPH
UNC SCHOOL OF MEDICINE
DEPARTMENT OF PEDIATRICS
CHAPEL HILL, NORTH CAROLINA

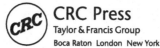

CRC Press
Taylor & Francis Group
Boca Raton London New York

CRC Press is an imprint of the
Taylor & Francis Group, an **informa** business

First published 2016 by SLACK Incorporated

Published 2024 by CRC Press
2385 NW Executive Center Drive, Suite 320, Boca Raton FL 33431

and by CRC Press
4 Park Square, Milton Park, Abingdon, Oxon, OX14 4RN

CRC Press is an imprint of Taylor & Francis Group, LLC

Library of Congress Cataloging-in-Publication Data

Steiner, Michael J. (Pediatrician), author.
  The little book of pediatrics : infants to teens and everything in between / Michael J. Steiner, Kelly Smith Kimple.
      p. ; cm.
  Includes bibliographical references and index.
  ISBN 978-1-61711-839-5 (alk. paper)
  I. Kimple, Kelly Smith, 1981- , author. II. Title.
  [DNLM: 1. Pediatrics. 2. Health Education. 3. Primary Health Care. WS 200]
  RJ48
  618.92--dc23

                                    2015029708

ISBN: 9781617118395 (pbk)
ISBN: 9781003524861 (ebk)

DOI: 10.1201/9781003524861

Illustrations by Jeff Moore.

Contents

vi   Contents ....

ACKNOWLEDGMENTS

I would like to acknowledge my parents, wife, children, brother, and other family members. Importantly for this book, my parents and wife have patiently helped to improve my writing at different stages of my life.

—*Michael J. Steiner, MD, MPH*

I would like to acknowledge the people that are home to me—my parents for laying a strong foundation, my husband for helping build a life together brick by brick, my son for bringing so much light, and to my sister for encouraging me to paint with brighter colors.

—*Kelly S. Kimple, MD, MPH*

We would like to also acknowledge all of our teachers, but particularly Wally Brown, MD. He has taught both of us a lot about general pediatrics and should particularly get credit for any practical and helpful knowledge in this book that is also fun.

—*Michael J. Steiner, MD, MPH*
and Kelly S. Kimple, MD, MPH

About the Authors

Michael J. Steiner MD, MPH, is a general pediatrician at North Carolina Children's Hospital and the University of North Carolina. He serves as the Division Director for General Pediatrics and Adolescent Medicine and the Director of Outreach and Network Development for the Department of Pediatrics. Previously, he has worked in a variety of settings from rural primary care to urban academic settings. He currently sees patients in primary care, a complex care referral clinic, hospitalized children, and in the newborn nursery. This is the first book he has co-authored, but has over 40 papers and chapters across a broad group of topics. He lives in Chapel Hill, North Carolina with his wife, two daughters, and an excitable dog.

Kelly S. Kimple, MD, MPH, is a general pediatrician at North Carolina Children's Hospital and the University of North Carolina. In addition to pediatrics, she has also completed training in preventive medicine and public health. She currently sees patients in primary care, a complex care referral clinic, a rural community health center, and in the newborn nursery. She lives in Chapel Hill, North Carolina with her wonderful husband, loving son, and a sweet but spoiled dog.

INTRODUCTION

We have both been lucky to have jobs where we care for children, help parents take care of children, and help others around us understand children a little bit better. Hopefully, in some small way, that work has helped to improve the lives of children.

One great thing about working with and for children is that it is incredibly rewarding and fun. Even the most serious moments can often have glimmers of light and levity. We hope this book helps people who work with children to understand some of the serious and important issues, while also sharing in some of the levity.

Sincerely,
Michael J. Steiner, MD, MPH
Kelly S. Kimple, MD, MPH

Chapter 1

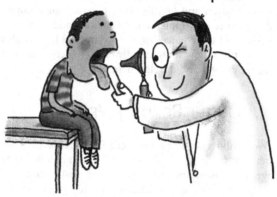

Just Checking In: Why Do You Need to "Check" on Well Children?

Kids, for the most part, are healthy, and prevention is a key component of pediatrics. So, why do these healthy children risk catching a cold in the waiting room to come to the clinic once in a while? The overall goals are

Steiner MJ, Kimple KS. *The Little Book of Pediatrics: Infants to Teens and Everything in Between* (pp 1-8).

to maintain physical, mental, and social health and to educate kids and their families. Even in the absence of illness, children and families may need encouragement and guidance to implement behaviors and activities that increase the chances of long-term health. It is also important to follow these rapidly changing children and optimize growth and development.

On the Road to Wellness

Well-child check-ups vary greatly because they are dependent on the age and needs of the child. Topics may range from discussions on infant care, breastfeeding, and immunizations to assuaging fears and feelings of inadequacy to awkward encounters with adolescents about the topics they least want to bring up with any adult, let alone their doctors (sometimes called the "sex, drugs, and rock-n-roll" discussion). These visits are the cornerstone of pediatrics supporting healthy growth and development. In addition to promoting physical and emotional health, providers can use this time to discuss any additional questions or concerns that the family may have.

The American Academy of Pediatrics and other groups provide guidance about what should be covered while clinicians try to keep children healthy. In 1990, the *Bright Futures* initiative, from the Maternal Child Health Bureau of the U.S. Department of Health and Human Services, was created to improve pediatric health services and offer standard recommendations for health care providers. These guidelines shed some light on making futures bright using widely applied tools and evidence-based strategies to improve the health of children. The *Bright Futures* Guidelines[1] facilitate the occasionally overwhelming task of keeping children healthy while also advocating for children, families, and communities. The recommendations for pediatric preventive health care are outlined by *Bright Futures* and followed by the Early and Periodic Screening, Diagnosis, and Treatment (EPSDT) program, a federal law that requires Medicaid to provide these recommended services.

Bright Futures proposes a standard schedule to get kids in for well-child checks. For high-risk or first-time parents, a prenatal visit can be a time to talk about what to expect, breastfeeding, and any other questions that might come up. The rapid growth and development of an infant necessitates more frequent visits, starting a few days after birth and then at 1, 2, 4, 6, 9, and 12 months. In early childhood, recommended visits occur at 15, 18, 24, and 30 months, 3 years, and then are spread out to yearly visits thereafter.

A well-child appointment can include the child's medical history; growth (including body mass index to assess for obesity) and blood pressure measurements; vision and hearing screenings; assessment of development and behaviors; a complete physical examination, including an oral health assessment; potential immunizations or laboratory tests, depending on age; and anticipatory guidance. We will go into more details on all of this later. These visits are an opportunity to screen individuals with no symptoms for particular conditions or determine the individual's risk of developing a disease, in addition to offering advice on healthy behaviors. Therefore, visits are packed full and there can be a lot to cover in a short time to promote child well-being.

SCREEN MACHINE

Because most of these children are well, they receive specified screening tests to look for problems before they develop. The idea is that if problems can be identified early or before they have symptoms, then early intervention can lead to improved long-term outcomes. Starting shortly after birth, the newborn screening program looks for diseases that can have serious and lasting effects on a child's health or even survival. Diseases such as phenylketonuria or hypothyroidism can be treated early by knowing the results from the newborn screening blood test to prevent detrimental developmental effects on the child. With genetic testing continuing to improve, the number of diseases that are included in the newborn screening program has increased, but which diseases are tested for varies by state.

Screening at each well-child visit depends on age and may include laboratory tests, standardized screening tools, or sensory screening. A 12 month old may need a blood draw for hemoglobin or hematocrit levels to check for anemia (decreased red blood cells in the body), or even a lead level if the child is at risk for lead toxicity. Sexually active adolescents should receive screening for sexually transmitted infections, such as chlamydia, gonorrhea, and HIV. Other tests, such as tuberculosis or cholesterol screening, may depend on the child's risk. Throughout childhood, providers also ensure that the senses stay sharp, with yearly vision and hearing screenings.

The next chapter will go into more detail on growth and development, but well-child visits are also a way to monitor that children are staying on track and to get assistance or services early to optimize development, if needed. This may include discussing developmental milestones with the family while observing the child or using more formal screening tools or standardized questionnaires. For example, the American Academy of Pediatrics and *Bright Futures* recommends screening for autism at 18 and 24 months using an approved screening tool because children have better outcomes if autism is diagnosed and treated earlier. The tool is usually a list of questions that the parent or guardian answers, giving the provider an objective way to determine whether there is a problem while also collecting more information. Beyond developmental concerns, emotional and behavioral screening is done in school-aged children and adolescents, including screening for depression or risky behaviors.

STICK IT

In addition to the occasional laboratory test or screening tool, a crucial part of maintaining child well-being is vaccinations. Although immunization programs are an incredible health achievement and have had a dramatic impact on decreasing or eradicating infectious diseases, getting a shot is probably the most feared part of these check-ups from the child's perspective. The Advisory Committee on Immunization Practices (ACIP), part of the Centers for Disease Control and Prevention (CDC), releases the recommended immunization schedule.[2] Although these are based on well-child visits, each visit to the clinic should be an opportunity to update any missing or delayed immunizations.

LET'S TALK

An important part of well-child visits that sets them apart from other visits is the concept of preventive service counseling and anticipatory guidance. This guidance targets keeping kids out of harm's way and staying healthy. The provider can have a discussion about what the family has been doing to promote health and expand on how to improve these behaviors. *Bright Futures* has a comprehensive list of topics to cover depending on age, although providers often prioritize based on the child's needs because it is difficult to cover everything at each visit. Topics for preventive service counseling can include injury prevention, safety, nutrition, physical activity, healthy behaviors, school performance, peer interaction, and avoiding risky behaviors. This also opens the door for counseling to change unhealthy behaviors, such as smoking cessation, or to promote healthy eating and physical activity for obesity. Anticipatory guidance is a type of preventive service counseling uniquely emphasized in the care of children where the provider, understanding development and common issues parents will face in the future, predicts what might become an issue for children before the next clinic visit and helps the family address health related to that change. For example, the provider might tell the family of a 10 month old that before the next visit, their child may start walking so they need to make sure that there is a gate at the top of their stairs now.

Injury is the number one cause of death in children and many of these injuries can be prevented. Providing a little information to the family targeted to the child's age makes a difference. The following are some of the recommendations health care providers make to families to prevent injuries:

- Car seat safety: the car seat should be rear facing in the backseat until age 2 years (or until the child outgrows it) and then a forward-facing car seat should be used. Once they outgrow the forward-facing car seat, a booster seat should be used until the child reaches the height that the seat belt fits properly (4 feet, 9 inches, usually between the ages of 8 and 12 years). Children should always ride in the back seat.
- Make sure home has working smoke and carbon monoxide detectors.
- Prevent burns by setting water heater < 120°F.
- Keep child away from hot liquids.

- Keep small objects away from babies because they are choking hazards.
- Never leave baby unattended in a bathtub or on high surfaces (eg, changing table, couch, beds).
- Lock up medicines, cleaning supplies, and any other hazardous material and write down the phone number for Poison Control. Lock up other harmful things, such as alcohol or scissors.
- Avoid walkers for babies.
- Put gates on all stairs.
- Do not have guns in the home; however, if you must, lock up the gun unloaded with ammunition stored separately from the gun.
- Stay within arm's reach of any child in or near water. Pools should be surrounded by fences.
- Protect that head with a bicycle helmet.
- Provide adult supervision for all play near roads or driveways.

THE VILLAGE

A lot happens to keep a well child healthy at these visits, but this health is not limited to the patient. A healthy environment is also crucial to optimize the physical, emotional, and social well-being of children, meaning that providers should also check in on the health of the family and community. For example, postpartum depression screening for the mother during infant visits can identify potential problems and provide an opportunity to improve both the mother's and baby's health. In addition, asking about interpersonal violence or neighborhood violence can give insight into the child's and family's situation, as well an opportunity to advocate on the family's behalf. The long-term health of children becomes largely dependent on the health of the family and of the neighborhood where they live, so the health care team also focuses on these issues.

Now, that is one big happy family...and child (minus the shots).

REFERENCES

1. American Academy of Pediatrics. Bright Futures. 2015. Available at: https://brightfutures.aap.org/Pages/default. aspx. Accessed August 28, 2015.

2. Centers for Disease Control and Prevention. CDC - Vaccines - Child, Adolescent, and Catchup Schedules for Providers. 2015. Available at: http://www.cdc.gov/vaccines/ schedules/hcp/child-adolescent.html. Accessed August 28, 2015.

Chapter 2

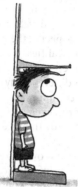

Keep on Growing (Growth and Development)

THE MEASUREMENTS

Measurement of growth is one of the core aspects of monitoring for health and wellness in children. It is uncommon for children who are growing, gaining weight, and developing normally to have a long-standing illness that has been undiagnosed. Conversely, abnormal

Steiner MJ, Kimple KS. *The Little Book of Pediatrics: Infants to Teens and Everything in Between* (pp 9-32).
© 2016 Taylor & Francis Group.

linear growth or height, head growth, and weight change can be early signs of diseases that otherwise have not shown other problems. Caring for children and families as brains and bodies are developing and changing dramatically is a unique aspect of the field of pediatrics compared with other medical fields. In children's health, the illnesses occur at different ages; the illnesses present or become apparent in different ways at different ages; the children or patients communicate differently at different ages; and treatments can even vary by age and as children grow. Some aspect of growth is measured at most doctor visits for children.

The most common growth parameter that is measured is the weight. For infants, scales allow the child to be placed in a small bassinet while lying down to calculate the weight in either kilograms or pounds. For older children, a digital standing scale can be used, as well as older scales that use a balancing of weights on top of the scale against how much the child weighs. Length is measured by laying infants and young children down on a table that is almost like a box where one edge of the box can be moved to the bottom of their feet while the top of their head is against the other edge of the box. Inches or centimeters are marked across the longer edge of the box to indicate the infant's length. Once children can stand and follow directions, something called a stadiometer is used to measure height. This tool is attached to the wall and children stand with their feet against the wall looking forward while a small bar is lowered to touch the top of the head. The attachment is scaled so that you can then read the height of the child based on the centimeters or inches that the perpendicular bar is above the floor.

Weight and length can be combined to calculate body mass index (BMI). The BMI attempts to normalize the weight based on the height of the child or demonstrate whether children are approximately the right weight based on their height. The BMI is calculated as the weight in kilograms divided by height in meters squared. For most adults, this produces a number between 18 and 35 kg/m². A BMI under 18 kg/m² is considered underweight, between 18 and 25 kg/m² is considered normal, between 26 and 30 kg/m² is considered overweight, and over 30 kg/m² is considered obese. Remember that children's body proportions change throughout childhood, so the absolute BMI number is not helpful. Instead, there are graphs that clinicians can use to show you where an individual child's BMI is compared to a sample of other children. Therefore, BMI in children is often reported as a BMI percentile or position within a larger group of children, where a BMI over the 85th percentile is considered overweight and over the 95th percentile is considered obese.

Head circumference is the last commonly obtained growth measurement in children, particularly in infants and young children. Although weight measures the amount of mass that is accumulating in the child and height measures the growth of bones, head circumference changes as the brain of infants and young children grows and pushes out against the skull that has not fully formed and therefore spreads out. For head circumference, a tape measure can be placed over the farthest point from the back of the head, or occiput, and wrapped around the head to the most forward part of the forehead. The circumference around the widest part of the head is used to measure head circumference. This is often the least accurate measurement, so ideally the same person should measure it each time to compare head circumference over time. Because it is fairly inaccurate, most people recommend taking three measurements and using the average of the three. There are other measurements of the body that can be taken, either of individual body parts, measures of fat on the body, or comparisons and proportions of the body, but height, weight, and

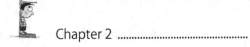
head circumference for young children are the most commonly used.

Clinicians should plot the height, weight, and, for young children, the head circumference on a graph that demonstrates usual growth patterns for children of similar ages. By doing this, they can not only determine the current percentile, but also monitor the growth velocity or change over time. Dramatic changes in growth velocity for any of these measurements are often the first sign of a medical problem. For example, a 7 year old whose height has gone from the 95th percentile to the 50th percentile over 2 years is concerning, even though the child still has an average height. Similarly, a newborn whose head circumference has changed from the 50th percentile at 4 months to the 95th percentile at the 6-month visit is concerning for increased pressure inside the brain, even though a head circumference at the 95th percentile may be totally normal for another baby. The standards used for charting growth are the World Health Organization (WHO) growth chart in children younger than age 2 years and the Centers for Disease Control and Prevention (CDC) growth chart for children aged 2 years or older.[1] The CDC growth charts are included in Figures 2-1 (A) and (B).

WHAT IS NORMAL LINEAR GROWTH?

Linear growth or height is a surrogate measurement for the growth of long bones in the body over time. During the first year of life after birth, length is largely determined by intrauterine factors, such as how good the placental blood supply was, whether there was adequate nutrition, and maternal genetic factors. An average birth length for a full-term baby is approximately 20 inches long, and by age 1 year an average length is approximately

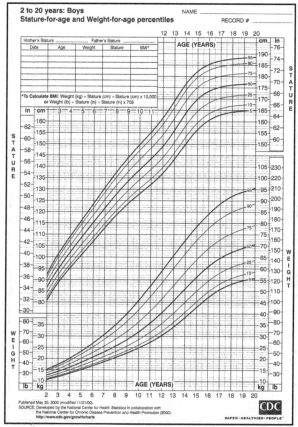

Figure 2-1A. Height and weight percentile curves for boys from age 2 to 20 years. (Reprinted with permission by the National Center for Health Statistics in collaboration with the National Center for Chronic Disease Prevention and Health Promotion [2000].)

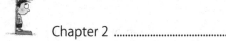

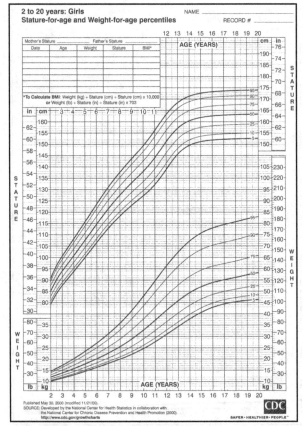

Figure 2-1B. Height and weight percentile curves for girls age 2 to 20 years. (Reprinted with permission by the National Center for Health Statistics in collaboration with the National Center for Chronic Disease Prevention and Health Promotion [2000].)

30 inches. Therefore, this is the time of most rapid linear growth, with a gain of 50% more height in 1 year.

During the second year of life, it is thought that paternal genetic factors begin to play a more important role in the linear growth rate and for this and other reasons many children become relatively taller or shorter compared to other children their age. Doctors describe this as crossing lines because of the lines on the growth charts at various growth percentiles: If a child starts at the 25th percentile of height at age 1 year and then grows more quickly than other children over the next year and is at the 75th percentile at age 2.5 years, then that child has crossed the 50th percentile line. Crossing percentiles can be normal in the first 3 years of life but, as you will see later, is not normal during school age.

Fun Facts: How tall will I be? There are multiple formulas that doctors can use to estimate eventual adult height. One of the simplest formulas is calculated by adding the mother's height and the father's height together, then if the child is a boy add 5 inches and if it's a girl subtract 5 inches, then divide by 2. This provides an estimate of the child's adult height. Sixty-seven percent of children will grow up to within 2 inches above or below this number and 97% will be 5 inches above or below. However, the equation is not quite as accurate if one or both parents are extremely short or if the parents' height was changed by something different than genetic potential, such as being short because of malnutrition during childhood or due to a severe disease during childhood.

School-aged children grow at a predictable rate of approximately 2.5 inches per year, and this is the same for both girls and boys. Because of this steady growth rate, children in this age range generally should not increase or decrease their percentile on the growth chart. Any major change, such as moving from the 50th percentile at age 6 years to the 20th percentile at age 8 years, should

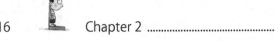

be closely considered by a physician and assumed to be due to a problem unless proven otherwise.

The final period of growth occurs during adolescence. This period of growth can be different from one child to the next, which is one reason you see such different heights in a seventh grade classroom. There is a range of ages that people go through normal puberty, and ages of puberty are different for boys and girls—girls generally grow early and boys generally grow late. You can see why such height differences show up! Let's examine each of these individually.

Girls can start puberty as early as age 7 or 8 years but averages are closer to age 10 years, with the first visual change being the start of breast budding. Girls start growing more quickly as this is developing and reach the maximum growth velocity just before the age when they begin menstruation. By age 16 years, most girls have completely stopped growing and reached their adult height. Male puberty starts later than in girls, with the first visual change being an increase in testicular and penis size at approximately age 11.5 years. Peak velocity of growth is also delayed, with an average age of about 14.5 years, which is about the time underarm hair growth begins. Although that is the time of fastest growth in adolescence, many boys will keep growing late into their teen years, but few boys grow after age 20 years.

WHAT IS NORMAL WEIGHT GAIN?

Weight gain changes at an increased velocity during the same periods that linear growth changes. At birth, common weights for full-term babies are between 6.5 and 7.75 lbs, but there can definitely be weights lower or higher than that in healthy babies. When born full-term, infants weighing less than 2.5 kg or 5.5 lbs are considered small for their gestational age, which can be due to just being smaller than usual but healthy or can be associated with insufficient nutrition, placental problems, maternal substance use, or various infections. Infants weighing more than 4 kg, or 8.75 lbs, are considered large for their gestational age. This usually is just a normal variation or genetics but can also be a sign of maternal diabetes during pregnancy.

Most breastfed babies lose weight after birth, sometimes up to 10% or 12% of their initial body weight. However, they then quickly gain it back, gaining an average of almost 1 ounce per day during the first 2 months of life and then two-thirds of an ounce during the next few months. Babies then often weigh more than 20 pounds by age 1 year, almost tripling their birthweight. This is the time of most rapid weight growth during life.

Similar to later in life, where BMI can adjust for the weight based on the height, there is a published curve that directly plots weight-for-length with percentiles to evaluate growth in the first 2 years of life. Children continue to gain weight through their teens, and unlike height growth, which has generally stopped by late teenage years, ongoing weight gain is considered normal. By age 20 years, healthy men will generally weigh 140 to 170 pounds, again determined largely based on height and body style, but in normal situations can continue to gain weight into the early 20s as the body takes on a fully adult shape and distribution.

UNDERWEIGHT AND FAILURE TO THRIVE

Some children do not gain weight normally after birth or during various periods in childhood. These children can become underweight, or be labeled as having "failure to thrive." Before weight or weight gain is labeled inadequate, the weight should be compared to average BMI, or weight-for-length in younger children, using those percentile curves. Sometimes, low weights can be normal for shortness or a small length, and if there is a problem it may be a problem of length growth instead of just weight gain. For children younger than age 2 years, a weight-for-length on the WHO curve greater than the 10th percentile with a normal weight growth rate or velocity suggests a normal weight for a given height. The same is true for a BMI greater than the 5th or 10th percentile if weight velocity is also normal.

The difficulty comes when the weight or weight-for-length is less than the third or fifth percentile or when there has been a period of weight gain that is slower than expected for age, causing the child to cross percentiles. Crossing percentile lines during the first year of life is common and by itself is not a cause for alarm. Similarly, by mathematical definition, approximately 5% of healthy young children will have a weight under the fifth percentile for their age. This is not true at older ages because the percentiles do not actually represent the current distribution of the weight in the population. Sometimes children with a weight-for-length under the fifth percentile, a weight under the fifth percentile, or weight percentiles that have crossed more than 2 major lines on growth chart will be labeled as having failure to thrive. In our opinion, this term should be abandoned because those are not definitive signs of any failure and the term has no standard meaning or definition. Instead, poor weight gain or low weight can be used to directly describe what is being observed. Children with low weight or poor weight gain often undergo evaluations for a medical cause of their weight change. Actually losing weight over a period of months during childhood is much more worrisome than a slow rate of weight gain because weight loss is uncommon but is a common signal of an underlying medical problem. In broad categories, weight loss or slow weight gain can be caused by inadequate caloric intake, not absorbing calories that are being taken in, or needing to use more calories than typical. Essentially, all causes of inadequate weight gain fall into one of these categories.

OVERWEIGHT

Although we often worry about poor weight gain, the most common weight gain problem for children in high-resource countries is now too much weight gain—or being overweight or obese. For infants, overweight is usually considered weight-for-lengths over the 95th percentile. The significance of being overweight in infancy is less well understood than later in life, although as you might expect, being overweight as an infant is a risk factor for being overweight later in life, particularly for infants who use formula. After age 2 years, BMI percentile is used to categorize weight status, with a BMI percentile ≥85th categorized as being overweight and a BMI percentile ≥95th categorized as being obese. Being overweight in early childhood usually does not cause immediate health concerns, unless there is severe obesity. However, as children age and as their overweight status becomes more extreme, they become more likely to have health problems related to their weight. In the long term, overweight children are likely to become overweight adults, and this is particularly true if their parents are overweight. Being overweight during adulthood is associated with and causes numerous health-related problems.

What causes children to be overweight? At a physiologic level, this is caused by taking in more calories than the body needs to use, arising from an incredibly complex interplay of changing caloric needs over time in childhood, multiple genetic factors, household habits, environmental issues such as advertising, food content, and food availability. It is rare for a medical condition or

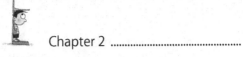

a simple single gene defect to cause children to be overweight, although diagnoses that cause obesity do exist.

DEVELOPMENT THROUGH CHILDHOOD

Physical growth is an important determinant of health
and is followed closely by clinicians during childhood.
However, another important aspect of growth and development is how the body is used—or how are the brain
and physical functioning developing? This is arguably
a more important sign of health and well-being than
physical growth.

Brain development and function are often tracked
across four broad categories. The first category is how
gross or large motor function is working. This measures
not only brain development, but also the function of
the musculoskeletal and nervous systems. An example
of a gross motor milestone is the ability to walk, and a
disease like cerebral palsy can affect gross motor development. In the second category, fine motor development
also measures brain development and musculoskeletal
function but in smaller muscle groups. This is linked
to gross motor development but also has some unique
individual aspects. Picking up small pieces of food is
an example of fine motor skill and can be difficult if
children have a tremor or a problem with balancing. In
the third category, language development measures how
children use speech, but we also monitor communication when speech is not used. For example, cooing is an
example of early speech formation and communication,
and children with brain injuries and autism can experience delayed speech. In the fourth category, how children
engage with their environment and interact with other
people develops in a certain consistent and predictable
way. For example, infants become scared of strangers

between age 9 and 12 months and they learn or master responding to their own name. Lack of those things happening can be a sign that something is not developing correctly in the brain.

THE FIRST YEAR OF LIFE

As is true for physical growth, the first year of life is a time of intense brain development and change in the being. At birth, babies have some temperament or personality but are largely guided by primal needs and innate reflexes. By age 1 year, children are starting to use words, are walking or moving around, and enjoy eating cake! Table 2-1 demonstrates the development of newborns across the 4 categories of development. An individual child can obviously vary somewhat in the age that milestones develop, and different spheres can develop at different speeds. However, the general pattern and approximate ages are also remarkably predictable in most environments.

AGES 1 TO 5 YEARS

Children in this age range begin developing their own personality and independence. A major milestone in this range is the ability to say "no," which often shocks and frustrates parents. The Terrible Twos are somewhat misnamed in that it is often the second half of the second year and the third year that are the most challenging, with a seemingly irrational ability to not do what the parent wants to happen. Table 2-1 demonstrates common developmental achievements during this age range.

Toilet training deserves special attention as a developmental stage for children, and a new step for parents.

Table 2-1
Infant and Child Development

Age	Social	Language	Gross Motor	Fine Motor
Birth	Can turn to mother's voice	Responds to sound, cries	Primitive reflexes guide some movements	Primitive reflexes, including sucking and grasping things in palms or on feet, hands fisted
2 months	Reciprocal smiling and responds to adult voice, social smiles	Coos	Chest up prone position, briefly steady head when held	Hands unfisted 50% of time
4 months	Smiles at pleasurable sights/sounds	Laughs out loud, vocalizes when alone	Rollover, sits if trunk supported, no head lag when pulled to sit	Clutches at clothes, reaches, plays with rattle

(continued)

Table 2-1
Infant and Child Development (continued)

Age	Social	Language	Gross Motor	Fine Motor
6 months	Reciprocation in babbling, smiles in mirror, stranger anxiety can start, stops momentarily to "No"	Duplication babble with consonants	Sits momentarily with propping	Transfers hand to hand, takes small objects, feeds crackers to self
9 months	Separation anxiety, orients to name	Uses sound to get attention, babbles and imitates wide range of sounds	Pulls to stand, crawls with all four limbs straight	Grasps with finger and thumb below
1 year of age	Knows name, cooperates in dressing	Says first words, points for communication, gestures (like waving)	Stands well with arms high and legs spread, some independent steps	Fine pincer grasp with finger and thumb, holds crayon

(continued)

Table 2-1
Infant and Child Development (continued)

Age	Social	Language	Gross Motor	Fine Motor
18 months	Engages in pretend play, shows possessiveness	Uses 10 to 25 words, points to simple body parts when named	Runs well, seats self in small chair, throws a ball	Can stack blocks, can draw a line or scribble
2 years	Plays next to other children but not with others	Uses 2 word sentences, uses > 50 words, 50% intelligible to stranger	Walks down stairs holding rail, kicks ball, and throws overhand	Imitates drawing a circle and horizontal line
3 years	Starts to share, fears imaginary things, and uses imagination to play	Uses 3 word sentences, uses > 200 words, 75% intelligible to stranger	Balances on 1 foot for 3 seconds, goes up stairs with alternating feet, rides tricycle	Copies circle, cuts with scissors, strings beads easily

(continued)

Table 2-1
Infant and Child Development (continued)

Age	Social	Language	Gross Motor	Fine Motor
4 years	Enjoys "tricking" others, has preferred friends, knows emotions like sadness and happiness	Words are all intelligible, although lisps or articulation errors are normal, uses 500 to 1000 words	Balances on 1 foot for at least 4 seconds, hops on 1 foot for 2 to 3 times, rides bike with training wheels	Copies square, ties a knot (maybe ties shoe), writes part of name
5 years	Has a group of friends, apologizes	Can define words that are simple, knows about 2000 words to use, responds to "why" questions, can rhyme	Walks down stairs alternating feet and no rail, balances on 1 foot for >8 seconds, can jump backward	Copies triangle, puts paperclip on papers, writes first name, spreads with knife

Children in different cultures begin volitionally voiding into a toilet at widely different ages, but there also is a physiologic component to when different children are ready to use the toilet instead of diapers. The median age for being toilet trained in the United States is about 33 months, but girls do toilet train slightly earlier than boys on average.[1] Accidents usually still happen in the months after toilet training is established. Ten percent to 15% of children will have occasional nocturnal enuresis (wetting the bed at night) even at age 5 years; however, daytime toileting should be well established before that for typically developing children.[2]

For children to toilet train, they generally have to be able to sense the urge to go, communicate the urge to go to an adult, have dry periods of time during the day, have a desire to be dry, have a desire to emulate older family members, and then have the motor skills needed to pull down their pants and diaper and to sit on a toilet. Again, despite these developmental needs, the age that typically developing children toilet train ranges from 18 months to 4 years in the United States.

It is generally recommended to follow a passive, or child-oriented, approach to toilet training. In this process, children are introduced to a small potty chair and encouraged to use it. Sometimes, parents put stool that was defecated into a diaper into the potty chair to get rid of it so that children realize that is where stool is supposed to go—and some children like to see stool flushed down the toilet. Parents should be warned that flushing scares some children, and often children do not like sitting dangling over the water. Successful toileting is praised, and accidents are acknowledged but never punished. Using this supportive and reinforcing method, toilet training often takes weeks to months once the child is able to achieve the underlying developmental skills listed above.

Fun Facts: Two developmental psychologists developed a "Train in a Day" method that involves encouraging the child to drink large volumes of juice or fluid and rewarding each toilet sitting with something like an M&M. This method has been widely used, although generally is not the endorsed method of pediatric professional societies.

THE SCHOOL-AGED CHILD (AGES 6 TO 11 YEARS)

Entering elementary school marks a new level of independence for children and their parents. This age range is often the start of sleepovers, homework, consistent sports participation, playing musical instruments, liking specific musical groups, gaining a sense of boyfriends and girlfriends, using a phone/computer/TV independently, and many other memorable aspects of childhood. This can also be a difficult time when school struggles and learning disabilities, anxiety disorders and attention deficit hyperactivity disorder, family instability and divorce, and other difficult childhood milestones or struggles can occur.

Erik Erickson was a famous psychoanalyst who is now best known for describing predictable patterns of development through childhood.[3] He described this period of time as being one where learning and creating become very active. He also emphasized the social development that occurs and the early positioning with peers that helps develop self-esteem and identity. This period also allows the later progression for adolescents to be focused primarily on friends and peers instead of parents and family.

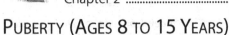

PUBERTY (AGES 8 TO 15 YEARS)

Puberty represents the start of a physical transformation from a child's body to an adult's body. In reality, physical development often continues into the late teens or early 20s, and with American adults' tendency to continue gaining weight through young and middle adulthood, the body habitus changes are almost never ending. However, that is not meant to decrease the emotional and physical importance of that first sign of breast development or start of pubic hair growth, both of which often shock children and parents. The timing of puberty is slightly different in boys than in girls and has a normal variation of years when it can start. However, there are some predictable timings and pace that are consistent within boys and girls.

The first sign of puberty for most girls is the development of breast tissue or breast buds, which will continue developing into adult breast structure. Actually, the first anatomic change is a change in ovary size due to the stimulation from the brain and a variety of hormones from the ovary and the adrenal glands that become active, producing the visible changes in the body shape and development. Regardless, breast development occurs at a mean age of approximately 10 years for all girls; however, interestingly Black girls' breast development tends to be earlier and can be as early as age 7 or 8 years, whereas European American or White girls tend to have later development.[4] Once some breast tissue has started to form, it is usually about another 2.5 years until menses starts, at an average age of just over age 12 years. Again, there is variation in this spacing and normal menses can start as late as age 15 years, depending on when breast development started. Girls' linear growth is the most rapid in the period of time immediately before menses, and most girls have stopped growing by age 16 years.

For some reason, female puberty has slowly been occurring earlier over the past 30 to 40 years.[5] It is not fully understood why that change is taking place.

For boys, the gonads or testicles are visible and can be easily examined (unlike the ovaries), so testicular growth is one of the first signs of puberty initiation in males. Boys generally begin puberty later than girls, with the average age of increase in testicular volume occurring at approximately age 11.5 years and pubic hair development starting around age 12 years.[4] The peak rate of height growth does not occur until about age 14 years, instead of age 12 years in girls. Sperm begin to appear at approximately age 14.5 years and pubic hair is fully developed by age 15 years for most boys. However, in males, physical growth often continues until age 18 years and strength, facial hair, and other results of puberty often continue into the early 20s.

ADOLESCENCE (AGES 12 TO 18 YEARS)

Adolescence is a time when normal development includes primary emotional connections to friends instead of family members and increased experimentation with pieces of adult living, including romantic relationships, first sexual relationships, possible illicit use of alcohol or illegal drugs, and jobs, driving, and other adult responsibilities. This age range can be a challenging time for parents but can also be full of great achievements and the realization of success based on the early years of parenting.

Physicians caring for children in this age range often focus on social and emotional development. This focus is validated by the epidemiologic statistics, which demonstrate that the 3 leading causes of death for adolescents are motor vehicle crashes, homicide, and suicide. A helpful pneumonic to explore the risk factors for those and

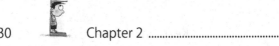

other causes of morbidity is the HEADSSS screening, or what some people refer to as BHEADSS:

B—Body image. How do teens feel about their body shape and size? This screens for anorexia and bulimia and creates the opportunity for discussion about obesity.

H—Home. What is the home like and with whom do they live?

E—Education and employment. What are their grades and school achievements?

A—Activities. What does the teen do for fun and entertainment? Significant connections and activities can decrease the risk of other risk factors.

D—Drugs. Screening for abuse of drugs.

S—Sexuality. Creates the opportunity for a discussion not only about sexual orientation, but also about safe sexual practices, which may help decrease the risk of infection or unintended pregnancy.

S—Suicide/Depression. One of the top three causes of death in this age range, there are validated screening tools for depression in adolescent patients.

Although much of the discussion about adolescents focuses on the risk factors and dangerous activities in which they can engage, there is also growing literature about things that help protect adolescents and maintain long-term healthy development. Some of the habits or situations that are associated with improved outcomes for adolescents and young adults are a regular family dinner, a tight connection with an adult in the home or in the community, participation in team sports, high achievement in school, clear occupational goals and a concrete understanding of the next step needed to achieve them, and opportunities to practice leadership and life skills. Although many of the studies of these behaviors in teens do not prove that each of these cause good outcomes, exposing an adolescent to these situations likely stimulates improved physical and mental health and increases the chance of becoming a healthy, balanced adult.

AUTONOMY AND THE FINAL STAGE OF CHILDHOOD AND YOUNG ADULTHOOD (AGES 18 TO 25 YEARS)

In this age range, children become young adults and can take widely divergent paths—from living with their parents and attending a local college (not that different than the teen years), to being in the Army and living in another country, to having their own job and own home without any parent involvement. We have learned a great deal in the past decade about brain development during this period of life, and we definitively know that young adults in this age range generally do not have fully formed adult decision-making styles and processes. Fully adult thought pattern develops around age 25 years, and then continues to be tempered thereafter by experience.[6] Despite this ongoing immaturity, most social systems officially consider individuals in this range to be adults—from the ability to obtain a driver's license, to the legal system, to the legal use of alcohol, to the ability to serve in the military, and to obtaining job and occupation opportunities. This traditional "graduation" to adult responsibilities with a still-developing brain sometimes causes problems. For example, this age range generally continues to have more impulsivity and risk taking behavior than do adults in their late 20s or 30s. This does not mix well with driving and legal use of alcohol, and the result is high rates of morbidity and mortality from motor vehicle crashes and alcohol-related complications.

During this stage, young adults often settle into a more balanced relationship with friends and families, with both playing important roles in their lives. Although most adolescents have had some romantic and sexual relationships prior to this age, this period may mark the first long-term romantic relationship, and, for many people, may lead to the initiation of marriage and/or having children of their own. For those who attend college or post-secondary education, this age range is usually the final period of formal schooling and education. In our society, by age 25 years, most people are settled into a track to their first occupation and are often taking responsibility for all of their essential daily needs, such as housing, food, health, and transportation.

REFERENCES

1. Centers for Disease Control and Prevention. Growth Charts. 2015. Available at: http://www.cdc.gov/vaccines/ schedules/hcp/child-adolescent.html. Accessed August 28, 2015

2. Howell DM, Wysocki K, Steiner MMJ. Toilet training. *Pediatr Rev.* 2010;31(6).

3. Erikson E, Erikson J. *The Life Cycle Completed.* New York, NY: W.W. Norton; 1998.

4. Sun S, Schubert C, Chumlea W et al. National estimates of the timing of sexual maturation and racial differences among US children. *Pediatrics.* 2002;110(5):911-919.

5. Euling S, Herman-Giddens M, Lee P, et al. Examination of US puberty-timing data from 1940 to 1994 for secular trends: panel findings. *Pediatrics.* 2008;121(Supplement):S172-S191.

6. News in Health. Teen Brains: Still Under Construction. http://newsinhealth.nih.gov/2005/september2005/ docs/01features_02.htm. Accessed August 25, 2015.

Chapter 3

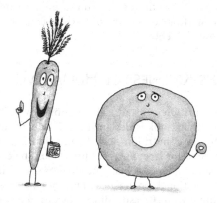

You Are What You Eat...and Drink (Nutrition)

Adequate nutrition is essential to the healthy growth and development of children. Some may remember the simple phrase, "An apple a day keeps the doctor away." And no, sugary apple-flavored cereals or apple juice do not count. Although many kids currently have a problem with obesity, which has highlighted the importance of good nutrition, it can be hard to know what children

Steiner MJ, Kimple KS. *The Little Book of Pediatrics: Infants to Teens and Everything in Between* (pp 33-46).
© 2016 Taylor & Francis Group.

should actually eat—not to mention how to deal with picky eaters. Food is essential but what one eats can be nutritious and healthy or sometimes even harmful to the body. Starting good nutrition early in childhood will have lifelong benefits.

THE KINDNESS OF HUMAN MILK

Good nutrition can start right after birth with breast-feeding. Human milk is designed specifically for infants and is the best nutrition—not to mention it is naturally provided for free. Breastfeeding should be encouraged for all mothers for many health reasons, including physical, emotional, or practical, but not all women are able to breastfeed. Breastfeeding provides better infant immunity, decreases infections, and likely decreases the risk of conditions such as diabetes, obesity, cancer, asthma, and sudden infant death syndrome. In addition, the mother benefits from a lower risk of postpartum depression, improved postpartum recovery, and lower risks of diabetes, ovarian cancer, and breast cancer. The American Academy of Pediatrics recommends exclusively breastfeeding until age 6 months and continued breast milk up until age 12 months, and even longer, if desired.[1]

Provided that the mother has an adequate and well-balanced diet, breast milk has everything an infant needs for the first 6 months of life, with the exception of vitamin D. Therefore, a vitamin D supplement is recommended for infants who are exclusively or mostly breastfeeding, starting within the first couple of months. Infants may not get the most iron from human milk, but full-term infants should not need iron supplementation and should have enough iron stored up to last them until 4 to 6 months, when iron-fortified cereal and other solid foods are introduced.

Fun Fact: Breastfed infants may gain weight more rapidly in the first 2 to 3 months of life than babies who are formula fed, after which weight gain then slows down—this can make it seem like breastfed babies are large in the first few months, but they have less risk of obesity as they get older.

For some infants, breastfeeding may not be possible or preferred and formula is an alternative. There are a variety of formulas on the market in different forms, including powders (to mix with water), concentrated liquids (to be mixed with water), or ready-to-use options (the easiest but most expensive option). There are also different compositions available, including specialized formulas for certain indications. Standard cow's milk–based formulas are appropriate for most full-term infants. Preterm infants require specialized formulas with extra calories and minerals. Other types of formulas include soy-based or hypoallergenic (protein hydrolysate, "predigested") formulas. Many are concerned that fussiness, gas, and colic may be related to cow's milk formula, but these are common problems that are often not related to formula. Occasionally, infants may have a true milk protein allergy and will require a hypoallergenic formula, which is easier to digest but is much more expensive. Soy-based formulas often do not help with milk allergies because infants who are allergic to cow's milk may also be allergic to soy milk. Soy-based formulas are lactose-free, but infants generally do not have difficulty digesting lactose unless temporarily (eg, after diarrheal illness) and do not require a soy-based formula. However, if the parent is vegan or if the infant has galactosemia (a rare disorder with an intolerance to galactose, usually tested by newborn screening), he or she may require a soy-based formula.

FUEL UP

Infants and children need more energy to keep up with all the impressive growth and development going on, especially in the first year of life. Following birth, infants have a slower start and can lose up to 10% of their birth weight (especially first-time breastfed infants), but then should be back up to birth weight by about 10 to 14 days of life. Typical full-term infants require about 100 to 120 kcal/kg/day, which they get from about 6 to 9 feedings over 24 hours. In general, infants take smaller and more frequent feedings due to their small stomachs (every 2 to 3 hours on average), but there is considerable variation among different infants, and breastfed infants in particular may prefer more frequent feedings compared to formula-fed infants. By about age 1 year, infants usually take about 4 to 5 feedings per day.

Around age 6 months, infants can start gradually exploring the world of food. Some may start as early as age 4 months. Most people begin with offering iron-fortified cereal, although there is no medical reason that food should be introduced in a specific order—except that iron-rich foods are good to introduce to breastfed infants because iron stores start to decrease between age 4 and 6 months. In general, a variety of food can be introduced and recent research is beginning to show that waiting to introduce certain foods may not be neces-sary.[2] It is good to start slow, introducing one new food every few days, and to introduce a variety of flavors and age-appropriate textures. Around age 9 months, infants are able to bring their hands to their mouths, so finger foods can be introduced, creating fun while learning to feed themselves. However, the food needs to be soft, cut into small pieces, and easy to swallow without chewing to prevent any choking. As the intake in solids foods increases, the amount of formula or breast milk required also decreases.

Around age 1 year, and after many messes at the table, infants are accustomed to a schedule of three meals per day with two to three snacks, although again, there can be a lot of variation. At age 1 year, infants can switch from formula or breast milk to whole cow's milk. However, if the mother would like to continue breastfeeding beyond age 1 year, she should be encouraged to do so. Introducing cow's milk before age 1 year may affect nutritional status given its differing nutrients, especially the risk of iron-deficiency anemia or even low calcium. Skim or 1% milk should not be used until age 2 years and most recommend whole milk given the need for fat at that age; however, given the prevalence of obesity, some providers recommend using 2% milk at age 1 year if the child is at risk. While transitioning to cow's milk, the child should also stop using a bottle and instead use a cup. Infants can start trying fruit juice if desired between age 6 months and 1 year, but infants and children should not have more than 4 ounces of juice per day.

It is normal for children older than age 1 year to not eat quite as much as he or she used to, mostly because they do not need as much nutrition for growth. Some children may seem like they temporarily lost interest in food. However, parents should not force-feed their children because this can cause ongoing behavioral problems related to feeding. In addition, children between age 1 and 2 years can be picky eaters and will express their dislikes. Families should continue to offer a variety of foods, and sometimes a child may even take a food that was previously refused. A balanced, healthy diet can be possible for toddlers, even if "balanced" occurs over the span of a few days.

After age 2 years, children mostly eat like the other members of their family. This is why it is important that the whole family eat a healthy, balanced diet. From the

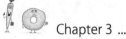

previous U.S. Department of Agriculture food pyramid that used to hang on walls of pediatric offices and schools to the more current MyPlate, visuals of good eating habits are beneficial for families to guide healthy eating choices. In general, kids should try to eat a balanced diet of fruits, vegetables, whole grains, low or nonfat dairy products, beans, fish, and lean meat. Junk food, including foods with saturated or trans fat and added sugar and salt, should be offered sparingly. Beverages can also be a large source of sugar and calories, so children should not be consistently given sugar-sweetened beverages and juice. Healthy foods can be difficult to obtain and can be expensive and, for many reasons, children who live in poverty or with food insecurity are actually more likely to be obese. See Table 3-1 for a rough estimate of how many calories children need at different ages, while taking into account a rough estimate of physical activity.

In children, a BMI between the 5th and 85th percentile is considered a healthy weight, a BMI between the 85th and 95th percentile is considered overweight, and a BMI above the 95th percentile is considered obese. The best weapon against obesity is prevention and calories from the diet should be balanced with physical activity to maintain healthy growth in children. Children should strive to get the recommended 60 minutes per day of physical activity or vigorous play. This does not mean spending an hour at the gym sweating on the elliptical machine or treadmill, but rather getting outside to run around, play, and expend energy. In addition, children are to limit the time in front of whichever screen of their choosing—television, computer (other than homework), iPad, iPhone—to less than 1 to 2 hours per day. This can be hard for kids, but screen time has been shown to be directly associated with obesity.

Fun Fact: The number 1 source of calories for children and adolescents is grain-based desserts, with pizza coming in at number 2 and sodas/sports drinks at number 3.[3]

Table 3-1
Estimated Caloric Need

	Age (years)	Sedentary	Moderately Active	Active
Child	2 to 3	1,000 to 1,200	1,000 to 1,400	1,000 to 1,400
Female	4 to 8	1,200 to 1,400	1,400 to 1,600	1,400 to 1,800
	9 to 13	1,400 to 1,600	1,600 to 2,000	1,800 to 2,200
	14 to 18	1,800	2,000	2,400
Male	4 to 8	1,200 to 1,400	1,400 to 1,600	1,600 to 2,000
	9 to 13	1,600 to 2,000	1,800 to 2,200	2,000 to 2,600
	14 to 18	2,000 to 2,400	2,400 to 2,800	2,800 to 3,200

*Adapted from *Dietary Guidelines for Americans, 2010*. Data are presented as averages. Sedentary is defined as typical day-to-day light physical activity. Moderately active is defined as typical day-to-day life, with physical activity equivalent to walking 1.5 to 3 miles per day (3 to 4 mph). Active is defined as typical day-to-day life, with physical activity equivalent to walking > 3 miles per day (3 to 4 mph).

We have been talking a lot about obesity, but now let us move on to nutritional deficiencies. Undernutrition and malnutrition can have a significant impact on growth and development (discussed more in Chapter 2). Even if a child has a specific deficiency, many times that same child is at risk for having other nutritional deficiencies. Severe undernutrition can range in severity and can be seen as a result of starvation, some unusual diet, or even chronic illness. *Marasmus* is the term for severe general nutritional deficiency and these children tend to look malnourished and emaciated and can have significant muscle wasting. *Kwashiorkor* is the term used for protein deficiency, and these children usually are thin with a protuberant belly, swelling, rash, and thin hair and can have a pale appearance. Many times there is overlap because protein deficiency occurs in conjunction with inadequate energy intake, so these deficiencies may not be two distinct conditions.

Providers may also have to consider nutritional deficiencies in children with specific disorders. For example, children with liver disease or cystic fibrosis have trouble absorbing fat-soluble vitamins A, D, E, and K. Kids on vegan diets or a breastfeeding infant of a vegan mother are at risk for vitamin B_{12} deficiency. Premature infants can be at risk for osteopenia (decreased bone density) or rickets (softening or weakening of bones) and need more calcium and phosphorus because these are poorly absorbed.

Isolated vitamin or mineral deficiencies can cause a variety of effects on the body and can be tedious to remember. Table 3-2 summarizes what happens when a person does not get enough, or perhaps gets too much, of a good thing. Many of the symptoms that occur are not commonly seen due to severe deficiency or toxicity rather than just not enough or a little too much.

Fun Fact: Even though it is good to have kids drink milk, iron deficiency anemia can be seen in toddlers who

Table 3-2
Vitamin and Mineral Deficiencies and Toxicities

Vitamin/Mineral	Not Enough	Too Much
Vitamin A	Trouble seeing at night, sensitivity to light, dry eyes, blindness, abnormal bone formation, defective tooth enamel, skin and mucus membrane changes, growth problems, increased infections, anemia, fetal abnormalities	Loss of appetite, slow growth, dry/cracking skin, liver and spleen enlargement, bone swelling and pain, bone fragility, increased intra-cranial pressure, hair loss, yellowing of skin, fetal abnormalities
Vitamin B$_1$ (thiamine)	Beriberi (disease affecting peripheral nervous system and/or heart), fatigue, irritability, memory trouble, loss of appetite, constipation, headache, insomnia, increased heart rate, inflammation of nerves, heart failure, swelling	None (if taken by mouth)

(continued)

Table 3-2
Vitamin and Mineral Deficiencies and Toxicities (continued)

Vitamin/Mineral	Not Enough	Too Much
Vitamin B₂ (riboflavin)	Ariboflavinosis (riboflavin deficiency with sore throat, swelling of mouth, magenta tongue, rash (seborrheic dermatitis), anemia, blurry vision, sensitivity to light, burning/itching eyes, poor growth, cheilosis (inflammation and cracking of the lips and corners of mouth)	None
Niacin (Vitamin B₃)	Pellagra (disorder of niacin deficiency) with 3 D's—diarrhea, dementia, dermatitis	Skin flushing and itching, liver problems
Pantothenic acid (Vitamin B₅)	Irritability, fatigue, numbness, stomach pain, vomiting, muscle cramps	Unknown, possibly diarrhea

(continued)

Table 3-2
Vitamin and Mineral Deficiencies and Toxicities (continued)

Vitamin/Mineral	Not Enough	Too Much
Vitamin B$_6$ (pyridoxine)	Irritability, seizures, anemia	Pain or numbness in hands/feet (only with high-dose supplements)
Biotin (Vitamin B$_7$)	Skin problems, rash	Unknown
Folic Acid (Vitamin B$_9$)	Anemia, mouth ulcers, tongue swelling, impaired immunity, neural tube defects in developing embryos (why pregnant women should take folic acid)	Unknown
Vitamin B$_{12}$ (cyanocobalamin)	Anemia	Unknown
Vitamin C	Scurvy: poor wound healing, bleeding gums, easy bruising, bone pain	Diarrhea, other gastrointestinal symptoms

(continued)

Table 3-2
Vitamin and Mineral Deficiencies and Toxicities (continued)

Vitamin/Mineral	Not Enough	Too Much
Vitamin D	Rickets (soft, weak bones leading to bone deformities), osteomalacia (softening of bones), low calcium (can lead to seizures)	Increased calcium that can cause vomiting, lack of appetite, pancreatitis, high blood pressure, heart arrhythmias, central nervous system effects, kidney stones, and kidney failure
Vitamin E	Neurological problems, anemia, impaired immunity, swelling of arms/legs, damage to retina of eye	Unknown
Vitamin K	Bleeding, bruising, problems with bone formation	Unknown
Calcium	Rickets, osteoporosis, numbness/tingling of fingers, muscle cramps, bleeding, emotional problems, seizures	Constipation, nausea/vomiting, loss of appetite, confusion, heart arrhythmias, kidney problems

(continued)

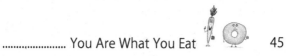

Table 3-2
Vitamin and Mineral Deficiencies and Toxicities (continued)

Vitamin/Mineral	Not Enough	Too Much
Phosphorus	Osteomalacia or rickets	Deposits in soft tissues, bone and heart problems, low calcium, bone pain
Fluoride	Dental caries	Discolored tooth enamel
Iodine	Hypothyroidism	Hypothyroidism and goiter (congenital hypothyroidism can occur from excess maternal iodine)
Iron	Anemia, decreased alertness, impaired learning	Nausea, vomiting, diarrhea, abdominal pain, hypotension, chronic excess → organ dysfunction
Zinc	Impaired growth, skin problems, decreased immunity, poor wound healing, diarrhea; acrodermatitis enteropathica is disorder from malabsorption of zinc	Abdominal pain, diarrhea, vomiting

drink a lot of milk. Children should not drink more than 3 cups (24 ounces) of milk per day!

REFERENCES

1. Breastfeeding and the use of human milk. *Pediatrics.* 2012;129(3):e827-841
2. Du Toit G, Roberts G, Sayre PH, et al. Randomized trial of peanut consumption in infants at risk for peanut allergy. *N Engl J Med.* 2015;372(9):803-813.
3. Reedy J, Krebs-Smith SM. Dietary sources of energy, solid fats, and added sugars among children and adolescents in the United States. *J Am Diet Assoc.* 2010;110(10):1477-1484.

Chapter 4

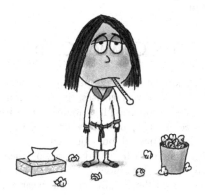

Sniffles, Sneezing, and Snot...Oh My! (Ears, Nose, and Throat)

Colds and viral respiratory infections are the most common reason for doctor visits for children, other than well-child check-ups. All children get colds and other viral infections. Occasionally, the viral infections

Steiner MJ, Kimple KS. *The Little Book of Pediatrics: Infants to Teens and Everything in Between* (pp 47-57).
© 2016 Taylor & Francis Group.

themselves can be serious, and even the common cold can develop complications, such as bacterial sinus or ear infections.

THE COMMON COLD

The common cold, or an upper respiratory infection, is caused by a variety of viruses, the most common of which is called *rhinovirus*. It is mainly caused by contact with secretions, particularly from direct contact, such as getting sneezed on, coughed on, or shaking hands with someone who has the virus on their hands. This is why people have now started to encourage others to sneeze into their elbow or even wear a mask in health care settings. Good hand hygiene is critical to help prevent infection, so hands should be washed frequently. As with adults, the common cold usually causes 4 to 10 days of nasal congestion, cough, low grade fever, and fatigue in children, and sometimes the cough can persist even longer.

Fun Fact: Children who attend daycare get more infections early in life, and sometimes seem like they are "always sick," especially during the first year of daycare. However, when they start kindergarten, they then have fewer missed days of school and fewer illnesses than children who never attended daycare.

Children usually get over colds without needing any other therapy. In fact, most over-the-counter medications for coughs and colds have never been shown to be effective any more than giving someone fake medicine or a placebo. These are a few therapies, some that have been around for centuries, that help with some symptoms:

1. Ibuprofen (for children older than age 6 months) or acetaminophen: These help with pain and

can decrease discomfort, including that caused by fever.

2. Honey: This treatment has been recommended for generations and has had a few randomized, placebo-controlled studies demonstrating that 1 to 2 teaspoons can help older children by decreasing cough.[1] Children younger than age 1 year should not eat raw honey because it can contain highly concentrated infectious spores called *Clostridium botulinum* and cause botulism, which generally does not occur from honey ingestion in adults. However, in older children, 1 to 2 teaspoons before bedtime can decrease symptoms of cough.

3. Mentholated rubs: Again, this works best for children older than age 2 years. There are case reports of complications due to use and problems with burns to the chest if they are put on and theoretically they decrease the function of the cilia in the airway, which helps clear mucus.[2] However, recent studies have suggested that they actually do decrease cough and cold symptoms and improve sleep while you have a cold.[3]

On top of some of these treatments, most people take it easy, get rest, and try to do things they enjoy while recovering from their illness; the same goes for kids!

ACUTE OTITIS MEDIA

An infection in the middle ear is caused by two things. The first is that the eustachian tube (the tube that drains the middle ear) stops working correctly. This often happens during colds due to swelling and inflammation, which prevents the tube from draining and ventilating the middle ear to the back of the throat. The "pop" you feel in your ear while going up a mountain or in an airplane is the tube opening to ventilate the middle ear and equalize the pressure in the middle ear with that in the air around you. In young children, the eustachian tube already has a tendency to not work very well, so colds make things even worse. When the eustachian tube stops working, pressure changes occur in the middle ear and fluid begins to accumulate. The second thing that has to happen to get a middle ear infection is that a virus or bacteria has to infect that fluid and begin to grow, which causes pressure to build up and causes pain. Most middle ear infections have both viruses and bacteria present in the fluid in the middle ear. Antibiotics can help shorten the length of illness in some children, but the most important treatment is aggressive treatment of the pain that ear infections cause.

SINUSITIS

Sinusitis is similar to ear infections in that drainage from the sinus is changed due to swelling or inflammation at the sinus openings (ostia) and fluid builds up. The fluid is usually infected by both viruses and bacteria, and swelling in the small spaces causes fullness and pain. Current guidelines recommend antibiotic treatment of acute sinusitis under certain situations, such as prolonged symptoms, cough from drainage in the throat that persists, or severe fever and facial pressure or swelling. Despite widespread use of antibiotics for sinusitis, at least some randomized, placebo-controlled trials have shown that antibiotics do not help shorten the symptoms for nonsevere sinusitis symptoms in children.[4]

ALLERGIC RHINITIS

Not everything that causes a runny nose is due to infections. Allergies are a common cause of a runny nose in children, especially in the spring and fall when environmental seasonal allergies strike. Allergies are an exaggerated response from a specific arm of the immune system. However, instead of protecting us from infections, this part of the immune system in affected people is overactive and actually causes the symptoms. The vessels in the nose get swollen and leaky and fluid goes into the interstitial tissue and the nose itself—causing the runny nose. The allergy that causes the nasal reaction can also trigger allergic reactions in the eyes, throat, lungs, and elsewhere, leading to other symptoms such as a sore throat or itchy watery eyes. These symptoms can be treated with anti-histamine medications, such as diphenhydramine, or newer antihistamines, such as loratidine or cetirizine. These medications prevent the release of histamine, which induces many of the symptoms that bother people during this time. Even more effective are direct topical steroid therapies, such as nasal inhaled steroids (eg, fluticasone or beclomethasone), and severe allergies are occasionally treated with oral steroids.

STREP THROAT

Strep throat is mainly an illness of school-aged children, although some children as young as age 3 to 4 years can get it. The primary and classic symptoms are (1) an exudate on the throat (whitish material on the throat and tonsils), (2) a fever, (3) anterior cervical adenopathy (enlarged, often painful lymph nodes on the front of the neck), and (4) lack of cough or runny nose. Younger children also often have abdominal pain and

Table 4-1
Common Causes of Sore Throat

Bacterial	Viruses	Irritants
Group A *Streptococcus*	Adenovirus	Drainage from allergies and nasal congestion
Mycoplasma pneumoniae	Coxsackie virus	Inhaling an irritant
Acanobacterium haemolyticum	Epstein-Barr virus	Yelling
Fusobacterium necrophorum	Influenza	
	Rhinovirus	
	Parainfluenza virus	

headache with strep throat infections. Strep throat is treated with antibiotics, usually penicillin or amoxicillin, to decrease the length of symptoms, prevent spread of the infection, and prevent complications, which include local extension of the infection behind the tonsils and rheumatic fever. Rheumatic fever involves an autoimmune (or one's own antibody) response to the bacteria that causes strep throat and can cause a variety of problems, including inflammation of the heart, lumps under the skin, uncontrollable rhythmic movements (known as *Sydenham's chorea*), and arthritis of a joint or joints. Thankfully, rheumatic fever is now rare in high resource countries due to strep throat treatment and changes to the bacteria that causes the infection. Strep throat is only one cause of sore throat and the many other common causes are summarized in Table 4-1.

INFLUENZA VIRUS

Influenza virus infection, or the flu, slowly circulates around the world and presents back in the United States every year at about the same time—when the air has started cooling off. As it moves around the globe, it undergoes changes to its genetic structure. These are usually minor changes (or antigenic drift), but a major change will sometimes occur, which is known as *antigenic shift*. These major shifts often lead to severe influenza seasons because the antibodies that people have from previous influenza infections can no longer help protect them from these dramatically different viruses. An example of a major antigenic shift occurred in The Great Influenza Pandemic of 1918, which lasted into the early 1920s, and estimates are that up to 5% of the world's population was killed by influenza.[5] A much milder influenza pandemic occurred in 2009 with another H1N1 influenza strain that people had not previously been exposed to.

In the United States, the flu often starts in the southwest and slowly makes its way across the country, being passed from one person to another. This usually happens sometime between October and March, but it only stays in one community for 6 to 10 weeks, and by then people have either been infected or are protected and it slowly decreases back to only sporadic influenza cases outside of the usual infection time. In most cases, young children, the elderly, and those with other medical problems are at the highest risk for severe influenza infection; however, there seemed to be particular risk with H1N1 infections to otherwise healthy people and pregnant women in 2009.[6]

In young children and infants, the flu often presents with fever, cough, breathing problems, vomiting, and diarrhea. In older children and adolescents, vomiting and diarrhea are less common, even though many people still ask, "Do you have the flu?" when people have vomiting and diarrhea. The classic presentation of flu in older children is high fever, cough, severe muscle aches, and fatigue. For otherwise healthy young people, a severe case of the flu is often remembered as the time they felt the most sick in their life. The treatments that help children with the flu include acetaminophen or ibuprofen if they have soreness or discomfort related to fever. It is important to not use aspirin in the treatment of children with febrile illnesses, except in specific rare instances where a doctor will prescribe it. We now have medications specifically targeted toward influenza viral infection, with oseltamivir being the most commonly used one for children. This medication helps to shorten the length of time children are sick with influenza, but only if it is taken within the first day or two from the start of infection. For children at high risk of complications, like those with breathing or other severe medical problems, or for those with severe infection needing treatment in the hospital, oseltamivir decreases the likelihood of complications from the flu, so treatment is given regardless of the duration of infection.

Remember, the flu is preventable. Most years, the flu vaccine is highly effective against the flu, but people have to be vaccinated every year—we do not yet have a vaccine that protects for multiple years. In addition, for children at a high risk of infection who cannot get the vaccine or those who just got the vaccine but the flu is already in their community, medication such as oseltamivir can also be used as a prophylaxis.

EPSTEIN-BARR VIRUS

Epstein-Barr virus (EBV) is the common cause of the "kissing disease," or mononucleosis, among older children and adolescents. Cytomegalovirus is a virus that can also cause a similar illness. Almost all children are exposed to EBV at some point in childhood and the majority of infections do not cause symptoms or only cause mild symptoms that are attributed to a common cold. However, the presentation that people usually think of with EBV is mononucleosis, which can occur in school-aged children, especially adolescents. This illness usually presents with malaise and a low-grade fever followed by a sore throat or pharyngitis, large painful lymph nodes in the front of the neck, and higher fever. This infection can be confused with strep throat or other infections. A secondary problem with this infection is that the spleen, an organ in the abdomen that is similar to a large lymph node and helps filter blood components, can enlarge just like the lymph nodes during this infection. When the spleen grows quickly, pressure is placed on the capsule of the spleen and, rarely, the spleen can rupture, which can be life threatening. Another unique aspect of the mononucleosis illness in adolescents is that it takes a long time to recover full strength and energy. At one time, it was thought that EBV caused people to develop chronic fatigue that lasts years, but EBV as the specific underlying cause of chronic fatigue syndrome has now been disproven.[7]

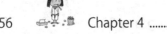

ULCERS IN THE MOUTH, THROAT, AND LIPS: HERPANGINA; HAND, FOOT, AND MOUTH DISEASE; AND HERPES SIMPLEX VIRUS

The Coxsackie virus, which causes herpangina and Hand, Foot, and Mouth disease, and the herpes virus are the usual etiologies of particularly difficult causes of a sore throat that includes painful ulcerations. These ulcerated areas can occur in the back of the throat, tongue, and lips, depending on the virus and presentation. When there is also a rash on the rest of the body, it can be called *Hand, Foot, and Mouth disease*, and as the name suggests, frequently includes macules or papules on the palms and feet and sometimes other places like the buttocks. The mainstay of treatment is pain control in addition to other treatments to support them and make them feel better. Some of the causes of sore throat in children, like Coxsackie virus infection, lead to ulcerations of the throat that are so sore children stop eating. These children sometimes need strong pain medications, or occasionally hospital admission, to provide them with intravenous fluids while their mouth ulcers heal.

REFERENCES

1. Cohen H, Rozen J, Krista H, et al. Effect of honey on nocturnal cough and sleep quality: a double-blind, randomized, placebo-controlled study. *Pediatrics*. 2012;80(6):150-151.
2. Mohapatra D, Friji M, Kumar S, Asokan A, Pandey S, Chittoria R. Camphor burns of the palm and non-suicidal self-injury: An uncommonly reported, but socially relevant issue. *Indian J Plast Surg*. 2014;47(2):252.

3. Paul I, Beiler J, King T, Clapp E, Vallati J, Berlin C. Vapor rub, petrolatum, and no treatment for children with nocturnal cough and cold symptoms. *Pediatrics.* 2010;126(6):1092-1099.

4. Garbutt J, Goldstein M, Gellman E, Shannon W, Littenberg B. A randomized, placebo-controlled trial of antimicrobial treatment for children with clinically diagnosed acute sinusitis. *Pediatrics.* 2001;107(4):619-625.

5. Taubenberger JK, Morens DM. 1918 Influenza: the mother of all pandemics. *Rev Biomed.* 2006;17:69-79.

6. Girard MP, Tam JS, Assossou OM, Kieny MP. The 2009 A (H1N1) influenza virus pandemic: A review. *Vaccine.* 2010;28(31):4895-4902.

7. Centers for Disease Control and Prevention. Chronic Fatigue Syndrome (CFS). 2015. Available at: http://www.cdc.gov/cfs/causes/index.html. Accessed August 25, 2015.

Chapter 5

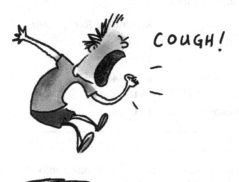

Take My Breath Away (Pulmonology)

If all that reading about colds and snot gave you a lingering cough, then you are ready for us to move down to the lungs. Coughing, wheezing, or even trouble breathing are all common pediatric problems with a long list of causes. We will not cover every pediatric pulmonary problem here but rather will attempt a general overview.

If a kid comes in coughing, it can seem obvious to think about the lungs, but many times it is not a

Steiner MJ, Kimple KS. *The Little Book of Pediatrics: Infants to Teens and Everything in Between* (pp 59-73).
© 2016 Taylor & Francis Group.

Table 5-1
Normal Respiratory Rate[1]

Age	Respiratory Rate (Breaths/Min)
Infant	30 to 60
Toddler	24 to 40
Preschooler	22 to 34
School-aged child	18 to 30
Adolescent	12 to 16

pulmonary problem (we will go more into this later). Physicians and other clinicians will note the type of cough in addition to other signs, such as how fast or how hard the child is breathing, the patient's color (warning: blue and dusky is not good), what the lungs sound like, and the oxygen saturation. All of these signs, along with a good and thorough history, are a start to figuring out what is going on.

DON'T HOLD YOUR BREATH

First, let's start with what is normal for breathing. The respiratory rate varies with age, starting with the fast breathing of a newborn to more of an adult pace in adolescence. How fast a patient is breathing may also be affected by things outside of the lungs; for example, fever or anxiety can increase the respiratory rate temporarily and sleep slows it down. Table 5-1 summarizes the normal respiratory rate for different ages.

THE AIR DOWN THERE

Children cough frequently and it can last for varying periods of time or come back repeatedly. Coughing can be acute or chronic, which can help narrow down the differential diagnosis at first. The most common cause of an acute cough in children is a viral respiratory tract infection, which was discussed in the previous chapter. The cough can come from irritation of the upper respiratory tract and postnasal drip, or the viral infection can also directly affect the lower airways and lungs. Most often, time and loving care are all that is needed for these viral infections, but it is not uncommon for the cough to linger longer than other symptoms, even up to 2 to 3 weeks.

Some infections, such as pneumonia or bronchiolitis, acutely cause coughing by directly affecting the lower respiratory tract. Lower respiratory tract infections tend to be more common in the fall and winter. Pneumonia is inflammation of the lung tissue and is most often caused by viral or bacterial infections, although it can also result from aspiration of food or other substances. Viruses, such as influenza, respiratory syncytial virus, parainfluenza, adenovirus, rhinovirus, and metapneumovirus, are a common cause of pneumonia, especially in young children. Children with viral or bacterial pneumonia usually have a few days of runny nose or congestion and fever (temperature may be a little higher in bacterial pneumonia). Tachypnea, or increased respiratory rate, and possibly harder breathing (using the belly muscles to breath or flaring nostrils), can be signs of a lower respiratory infection, as well as low oxygen saturation levels. Oxygen saturations measure the percentage of hemoglobin on red blood cells in the arteries that are saturated with oxygen. This is a measure of the amount of oxygen available for the body to use and for otherwise healthy people ranges from 97% to 100%. Older children may show signs of pneumonia with a high fever, chest pain, and cough. Abnormal sounds (snap, crackle, pop) can be heard with a stethoscope over the affected part of the lung and a chest x-ray can also be used to visualize abnormalities of the lungs.

There is an increased risk of bacterial pneumonia in children who are not fully immunized or in those children predisposed to bacterial infection from some viral infections. In those children with community-acquired pneumonia, the following are the most common bacterial causes: *Streptococcus pneumoniae, Chlamydophila pneumonia*, and *Mycoplasma pneumoniae. S pneumoniae, Staphylococcus aureus*, and *Streptococcus pyogenes* are causes of pneumonia in hospitalized children. Atypical pneumonia, caused by *C pneumoniae* or *M pneumoniae*, has an atypical, usually less severe presentation and is most commonly seen in older children or adolescents with low-grade fever and patchy areas observed on chest x-ray. Other infectious causes should be considered, especially in immunocompromised children or those with lung disease, such as cystic fibrosis. We have mentioned the most common causes of pneumonia, but Table 5-2 summarizes the many possible etiologies, including bacteria, viruses and even fungi and other uncommon causes. Appropriate antibiotic therapy is needed for the treatment of bacterial pneumonia, although it is unclear how much antibiotic treatment helps with atypical pneumonias. Sometimes hospitalization is necessary if blood oxygen level is low, if there is respiratory distress or an inability to take medications, or if close monitoring is required.

Some viruses can affect the lungs and lead to an infectious syndrome called *bronchiolitis*, which is an acute disorder of the lower respiratory tract and is a frequent cause of hospitalizations among infants. This infection typically causes swelling and fluid to accumulate in the small airways of the lungs and can lead to wheezing in

Table 5-2
More Causes of Pneumonia Than You Ever Wanted to Know

Bacterial	Viral	Fungal	Other
Streptococcus pneumoniae	Respiratory syncytial virus	Histoplasma capsulatum	Coxiella burnetii
Group B streptococcus	Parainfluenza types 1 to 3	Cryptococcus neoformans	Rickettsia rickettsii
Group A streptococcus	Influenza A, B	Aspergillus species	Mycobacterium tuberculosis
Mycoplasma pneumoniae	Adenovirus	Mucormycosis	Mycobacterium avium-intracellulare
Chlamydophila pneumoniae	Metapneumovirus	Coccidioides immitis	Pneumocystis jiroveci
Chlamydia trachomatis	Rhinovirus	Blastomyces dermatitidis	Eosinophilic (Ascaris, Strongyloides, other parasites)

(continued)

COUGH!

Table 5-2
More Causes of Pneumonia Than You Ever Wanted to Know (continued)

Bacterial	Viral	Fungal	Other
Mixed anaerobic bacterial infections	Enterovirus		
Gram negative enteric bacteria	Herpes simplex virus		
Haemophilus influenzae	Cytomegalovirus		
Staphylococcus aureus	Measles		
Moraxella catarrhalis	Varicella		
Neisseria meningitidis	Hantavirus		
Francisella tularensis	SARS coronavirus		
Nocardia species			
Chlamydophila psittaci			
Yersinia pestis			
Legionella species			

infants and small children from narrowing of airways, in addition to trouble breathing and low oxygen saturation. Chest x-ray can show patchy areas of infection, areas of airway collapse (atelectasis), or overinflated lungs. Currently, providers may do viral laboratory testing to aid in diagnosis. Treatment is mainly supportive, such as providing extra oxygen and intravenous fluids.

Respiratory syncytial virus (RSV) is a specific type of viral infection that can range from no symptoms or a very mild cold to children not being able to breathe for themselves and being put on a ventilator. RSV causes more than half of the cases of bronchiolitis, but bronchiolitis can occur from other viruses, such as metapneumovirus, parainfluenza, or influenza. Many times, an infant is exposed to someone with a cold and experiences a few days with a runny nose, decreased appetite, and fever. Fortunately, the majority of infections from this virus are mild and almost all children have been exposed to this by the time they are age 2 years. However, infants who were born prematurely (especially extremely premature infants like those born at 24 or 26 weeks gestation instead of the full 40 weeks), those with underlying lung problems, or those with serious heart problems are at especially high risk from this infection. These children might qualify to take palivizumab, an antibody that helps protect against RSV and slightly decreases the risk of severe infection in the first 2 years of life. This injection is expensive and needs to be given monthly during the time of year when RSV is circulating in the local population.

When RSV affects the lungs, it usually involves most of the two lungs, and therefore can cause the oxygen levels in the blood of infants to decrease and difficulty breathing and eating. For children with moderately severe RSV infection, these are the most common problems, and sometimes lead to children getting admitted to the hospital to receive intravenous fluids, oxygen to help support breathing, and rest. The difficulty oxygenating and breathing can be due to fluid or debris in the small airways and narrowing of the airways and from small segments of the airway collapsing, which is called *atelectasis*. All of these things can cause abnormalities on x-rays that can be confused with bacterial pneumonia. For this reason, children with bronchiolitis are sometimes mistakenly treated for bacterial pneumonia. Both are infections of the lower respiratory tract, but bronchiolitis does not improve with antibiotics. RSV is also a common cause of ear infections, so the children have pain and a fever on top of the difficulty breathing and eating—an all-around miserable few days. A particularly scary part of RSV infection is that early in the infection, particularly in premature infants, children can have periods where they stop breathing or have apnea. This always needs monitoring and support in the hospital if it happens.

We do not have a good treatment for bronchiolitis or RSV infection. As discussed previously, children with more severe disease often need to be admitted to the hospital for extra oxygen, fluids, and close monitoring. For the most severe cases of bronchiolitis, children will have a breathing tube inserted into the airway and be placed on a ventilator. Other treatments currently being investigated include having the children inhale salty nebulized water to dry up the airways and having children go home from the hospital while still using a little oxygen for a few days to 1 week.[2] Other medications have been tried and are generally thought not to help, including oral steroid medications and albuterol, which are used for asthma. The cough and breathing difficulties from RSV can last weeks after the initial infection and may make children more likely to have episodes of wheezing or other lung problems during the rest of infancy and toddlerhood.

BLOWING BACK AROUND

For a recurrent or persistent cough, the most common cause in children is asthma, or reactive airway disease. Asthma is a common chronic disease in children and is responsible for many pediatric office appointments, emergency department visits, and even hospitalizations. Chronic and acute inflammation of the lungs and restriction of the airways leads to symptoms such as cough, chest tightness, trouble breathing, and wheezing. Wheezing is heard with a stethoscope placed over the lungs and is a sign of lower respiratory tract obstruction and can be present with diseases other than asthma. The cause of asthma is not completely clear but seems to be a combination of genetic risk and an immune response to environmental exposures. Risk factors that might suggest asthma as a cause of cough or wheeze include allergic rhinitis, eczema, food allergies, family history of asthma, or isolated symptoms not associated with a cold.

Lung function tests can be used to confirm asthma or assess control of asthma symptoms. Children younger than age 5 years usually cannot do lung function testing because they have to follow instructions and take deep breaths into a mouthpiece. The test measures airflow to see how the lungs take in air, how air is released, and how quickly it is released. This creates a flow diagram, in addition to specific lung measurements, that are helpful in diagnosing any obstruction or restriction in lung function. For asthma, a bronchodilator such as albuterol can be given between tests to assess for improvement, which supports a diagnosis of asthma.

Some children will have recurrent wheezing that is related to a viral upper respiratory tract infection. These children do not always grow up to have asthma. On the other hand, children with allergies and asthma may have problems that persist into adulthood. Treatment of asthma depends on severity but includes avoiding any triggers, decreasing inflammation with daily, inhaled steroid medication, use of a quick-relief inhaled bronchodilator such as albuterol for asthma attacks, and occasionally a course of oral steroids for more severe exacerbations.

Other causes of chronic or recurrent cough that can look like asthma include gastroesophageal reflux and chronic sinusitis. These are not always obvious in children because they may not report the typical symptoms other than a cough. In addition, kids may have one of these problems in addition to asthma, which makes controlling asthma symptoms harder if these problems are not identified and managed. Young children are always putting things in their mouths, so foreign body aspiration should always be considered, especially if symptoms come on suddenly without viral symptoms (choking is not always witnessed). In addition, a habit cough (otherwise known as a "psychogenic cough" or a "tic") can be the cause of a cough lasting for weeks or months without response to treatment. This cough gets better while sleeping or even with a little distraction. There is an extensive list of possible causes of chronic or recurrent cough, so we will not cover everything, but Table 5-3 provides an overview.

Pertussis, or whooping cough, deserves to be mentioned because it has made a comeback due to inadequate or waning immunization. It is a highly contagious illness caused by the bacterium *Bordetella pertussis* that only uses humans as hosts. After being infected with the bacteria, there is usually about 1 week where the bacteria grows silently and then the child will develop cold symptoms such as a runny nose, mild fever, and cough for about 1 week. However, instead of getting better, the cough starts to intensify, leading to intense paroxysms of cough or coughing fits that make it difficult to breath. As the child tries to catch his or her breath, he or she often takes a deep breath in, which causes the "whoop" of

Table 5-3
Causes of Recurrent or Chronic Cough

- Asthma/reactive airways
- Postnasal drainage from upper airways
- Aspiration syndromes, recurrent aspiration (cleft or tracheoesophageal fistula)
- Frequent recurrent respiratory tract infections
- Chronic sinusitis
- Foreign body aspiration
- Gastroesophageal reflux
- Hypersensitivity following infection
- Bronchitis or tracheitis
- Idiopathic pulmonary hemosiderosis
- Bronchiectasis (cystic fibrosis, primary ciliary dyskinesia, immunodeficiency)
- Pertussis (whooping cough)
- Compression of the respiratory tract (vascular ring, neoplasm, lymph node, or cyst)
- Tracheomalacia or bronchomalacia
- Tumors
- Tuberculosis
- Habit cough
- Hypersensitivity pneumonitis
- Fungal infections
- Inhaled irritants (ie, tobacco smoke)
- Irritation of external auditory canal

whooping cough. This period of episodic coughing can last up to 3 months for some children before it goes away.

In older children and adults, this disease is annoying and bothersome; however, infants with pertussis experience feeding difficulty, gagging, and low oxygen levels and can even have apnea, or actually stop breathing, due to the infection. It is important to note that many

infants do not have a whoop during whooping cough
infection. With the severe symptoms in infants and
the risk of another bacterial infection occurring with
pertussis, infants can die from whooping cough. Sadly,
most infants get whooping cough from someone in
their household. A small percentage of adolescents and
adults with a cough that lasts longer than 2 weeks may
be infected with pertussis. This can easily be transmitted
to infants and young children. Luckily, pertussis vaccination has helped to greatly reduce pertussis infection rates
since the 1950s. However, pertussis vaccination as an
infant does not provide 100% protection and protection
wanes over time. For this reason, a booster tetanus vaccination as an adolescent or adult now includes pertussis
vaccination to provide improved protection. Vaccination
protects most people who get it, and the illness is often
much milder for those who are infected despite vaccination. However, because newborn babies and young
infants cannot be fully vaccinated immediately, it is
important that parents and those people around them
get a pertussis booster to protect them after birth. This is
also why it is recommended that women get vaccinated
during pregnancy to protect the newborn. Unfortunately,
recent decreases in immunization rates in some communities have led to pertussis outbreaks and epidemics and
the overall pertussis infection rate in the United States
has been increasing.

Most newborns and young infants with a diagnosis
of pertussis are hospitalized for observation and assistance with feeding and to assure they can be treated
quickly if they develop apnea. Older children only are
hospitalized if their oxygen level becomes dangerously
low during coughing or if they cannot consistently eat
or drink. Once children have severe cough symptoms,
antibiotics do not really help treat the disease but rather
help to prevent transmission to other children or family

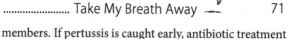

members. If pertussis is caught early, antibiotic treatment can shorten the course and make the illness less severe.

Fun Fact: Whooping cough is sometimes called the "100 days' cough" or the "cough of 100 days." Now that is a prolonged cough!

Tuberculosis is an infection of the lungs (but can infect other organs) caused by *Mycobacterium tuberculosis*. This infection is uncommon in the United States but is common in some other countries and is a serious illness when people get it. It is spread by inhaling respiratory droplets (picture a juicy sneeze or cough) from an infected person. Tuberculosis can be a cause of prolonged or chronic cough sometimes associated with fever, night sweats, and weight loss. However, there are people with latent tuberculosis who do not have any symptoms. It is important to ask about risk factors, such as contact with an infected person, immigration, travel to certain countries, or contact with incarcerated individuals. If the child is at risk, even without symptoms, then a tuberculin skin test (purified protein derivative or PPD) should be performed.

Fun Fact: Individuals who have received the bacilli Calmette-Guerin vaccination in other countries may have a falsely positive tuberculin skin test. We now have a blood test that can help differentiate whether people have a positive skin test from vaccination or from actual exposure.

STRIDE ON WITH STRIDOR

After all of the talk about coughing, wheezing, and whooping, let's move on to another sound—stridor. Stridor is a high-pitched sound upon breathing in that can be a sign of upper airway obstruction. There are multiple causes of stridor, but the most common in children is an illness called *croup*, which causes a barking cough and stridor predominantly in kids between age 6 months and 4 years. The "croupy" or bark-like cough of croup is one of the most recognized infections of childhood. Croup usually refers to a viral infection of the respiratory tract with swelling around the vocal cords, also known as laryngotracheobronchitis (which is why people usually just call it croup). Swelling can also involve the vocal cords, giving children a raspy or hoarse voice. The syndrome of this infection is often a fever, runny nose, and cough that develops relatively quickly and is worse at night. On examination, the lungs often sound clear with a stethoscope, but you can hear turbulent air movement or a whirring if you listen over their throat or sometimes you can hear a little squeak when they take a deep breath in. The barky, seal-like cough is almost pathognomonic. However, remember that asthma can sometimes produce a similar sounding cough, especially in young children, as well as anything that partially blocks the airway. Always make sure there is no way the young child swallowed a toy or got something stuck in his or her throat before you assume that sound is from croup!

Mild cases of croup will get better on their own after 2 to 3 days. For more severe or bothersome cases, oral steroid medications work to decrease the swelling in the upper airway, and the infection is usually waning by the time a longer-acting steroid wears off. For acute difficulty breathing from the swelling, inhaled epinephrine helps decrease the swelling in that part of the airway by making the blood vessels contract. Stridor and trouble breathing get worse when the child is upset, so it is a good idea to try and avoid things that make him or her mad (like a lot of things done in the clinic when you think about it—might take some extra effort). Antibiotics do not help treat this viral infection unless there is some other type of infection occurring at the same time. There are some children that get "recurrent croup" or "spasmodic croup" that may have an allergic component, but we will not go into that here.

Now, are you breathless with all that information?

Fun fact: Why do coughs get worse at night? It is not completely known why many types of coughs seem worse at night. Reasons that might play a role include that you focus more on it as you are trying to sleep or do other quiet things, parents are home with their children and therefore hear it, and the air gets cooler. However, one explanation that is known to be true is that overall breathing is slightly worse at night in everyone. There is likely some circadian rhythm to your lung function, and you do not usually notice any difference because you are not trying to use your full lung function at night. This has even been studied in nighttime workers, who continue to demonstrate slightly decreased pulmonary function testing at night—even though that is when they are awake the most. When you have an asthma attack or some other breathing problem, this slight difference becomes much more important and likely contributes to some of the worsening cough at night.

Reference

1. Ralston M. *PALS Provider Manual.* Dallas, TX: American Heart Association; 2006.
2. Zhang L, Mendoza-Sassi RA, Wainwright C, Klassen TP. Nebulised hypertonic saline solution for acute bronchiolitis in infants. *Cochrane Database Syst Rev.* 2013;31;7:CD006458.

Chapter 6

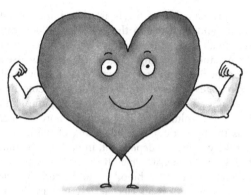

Pump It Up
(Cardiovascular)

Heart disease is a common cause of morbidity and death among adults in the United States but is not a common problem in children. However, when cardiac problems are present in children, they can be dangerous and life threatening. This chapter will review the structure of the normal heart and the most dangerous congenital heart problems, and then discuss murmurs, chest pain, and fainting, which often worry parents as their children get older.

Steiner MJ, Kimple KS. *The Little Book of Pediatrics: Infants to Teens and Everything in Between* (pp 75-90).
© 2016 Taylor & Francis Group.

THE HEART OF THE PERSON

The primary role of the heart is to pump blood to the lungs and then out to the body. The blood carries oxygen to all parts of the body, as well as other essential nutrients, and circulating oxygenated blood is essential for life. The heart can partially vary the amount of blood that circulates either by pumping or squeezing harder (the volume of blood increases with each pump, known as the stroke volume) or by pumping more frequently (this is the heart rate). The squeezing of the heart and the stroke volume are dependent, in part, on the muscle in the left ventricle, which is the strongest part of the heart muscle and pushes blood out to the body. The heart rate is dependent on an electrical system in the heart that coordinates and regulates the speed of contraction through the heart. Therefore, the amount of blood that circulates, or cardiac output, is a result of the heart rate and the stroke volume. Younger children are better able to increase their cardiac output as needed by increasing their heart rate, although both variables do change.

When the fetus is inside the womb, their circulation is partially based on their own heart pumping and partially dependent on the mother's circulation (Figure 6-1). In the first 48 to 72 hours after birth, a series of events normally happens that switches the fetus from fetal circulation partially using the mother to the functioning of the heart and vessels similar to an adult. These events start when the baby takes their first deep breath in and the umbilical cord is cut and more blood starts flowing to the lungs, and later the ductus arteriosus, which connected the pulmonary artery to the aorta, closes. This coordinated series of events happens with remarkable fidelity but not 100% of the time. Sometimes the anatomy is normal in the infant, but the full transition to adult circulation (Figure 6-2) does not happen. For example,

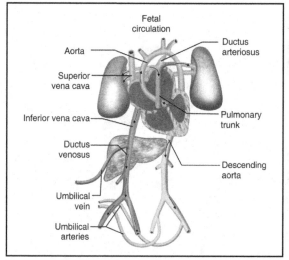

Figure 6-1. Fetal circulation.

occasionally the ductus arteriosus does not close off completely and continues to leak blood. Other times, the normal sequence of events does not happen because there is an anatomic problem with how the heart has developed. This is called *congenital heart disease*.

An evaluation of the heart is done during physical examinations. First, the child's general appearance and color is partially dependent on heart function. Second, doctors should examine the pulse in the legs and arms, particularly to identify some of the problems that occur with congenital heart disease. Doctors for children should also take a blood pressure measurement in infants if there are suspected problems or start taking blood pressures in older kids to screen for elevated levels. Sometimes doctors will lay their hand on the chest to feel the heart beating, but all health care providers will listen

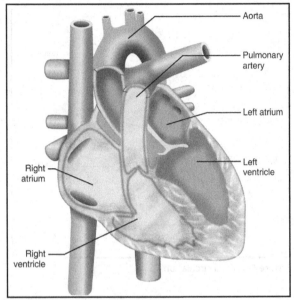

Figure 6-2. Normal heart anatomy.

to the heart beat at most examinations. When doctors listen to the heart, they can hear the speed at which it is beating, the regularity of the beating, the sounds generated when heart valves close (this is actually the beat heard when listening), and whether blood is moving around the heart or the vessels near the heart. This last sound is called a *murmur* or *heart murmur*. As the name implies, many heart murmurs are quiet and one must concentrate to hear them. Most heart murmurs heard in children are totally normal and not a sign of any heart problem. In fact, it is likely that all children have a murmur that can be heard at some point in childhood if the right person is listening at the right time. It is particularly common to hear murmurs at sick visits when children

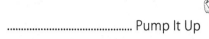

have fevers or do not feel good for some other reason and their heart is working a little bit harder to increase the cardiac output; murmurs can also be more common at certain ages. Occasionally, a murmur or some other part of the cardiac examination will have certain characteristics that make the clinician concerned that it may be a sign of a structural problem with the heart. In these cases, your clinician would either refer the child to a pediatric cardiologist for further evaluation or they might order an echocardiogram, which is an ultrasound of the heart. Echocardiograms are the primary way that structural problems with the heart are detected in children. An electrocardiogram is the primary way that problems with the electrical conducting system and heart rhythm or rate are detected. There are more specialized tests of heart structure and heart rhythm that are usually only ordered by cardiology specialists.

PROBLEMS WITH THE PLUMBING

Congenital heart disease can be broken into two categories: cyanotic or non-cyanotic. Basically, cyanotic congenital heart disease means that a problem develops with the oxygenation of the blood and the shifting of blood from the lungs (where it gains oxygen) to the body (where oxygen is used). Non-cyanotic congenital heart disease is a kind of heart problem that does not necessarily decrease the level of oxygen, but there is some other change from the usual heart structure.

Two of the more common heart defects are atrial septal defect (ASD) (Figure 6-3) and ventricular septal defect (VSD) (Figure 6-4). These occur when a hole fails to close during the development of the heart. An ASD allows blood to leak between the left and right atrium. A VSD allows blood to move directly between the left and right ventricle. Because the pressure in the left

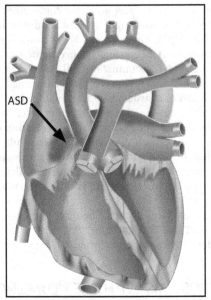

Figure 6-3. Atrial septal defect.

ventricle is normally much higher than pressure in the right ventricle, blood moves quickly between them, often causing an abnormal sounding heart murmur.

There are five main types of cyanotic congenital heart disease: truncus arteriosus (Figure 6-5), transposition of the great vessels (Figure 6-6), tricuspid atresia, Tetralogy of Fallot, and total anomalous pulmonary venous return (Figure 6-7). Each of these problems becomes apparent at slightly different ages, but generally they are detected either by ultrasounds during pregnancy or in the first hours to months of life. They each have unique traits that lead to the diagnosis and prognosis varies based on both the diagnosis and specific unique characteristics of the infant. However, they are all serious heart problems that

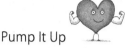

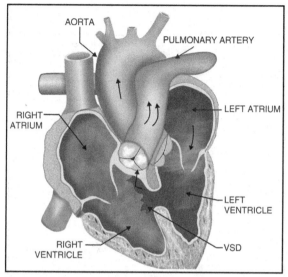

Figure 6-4. Ventricular septal defect.

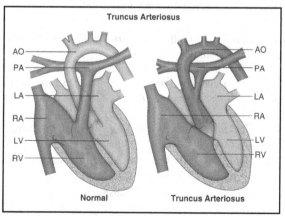

Figure 6-5. Truncus arteriosus.

Chapter 6 ....

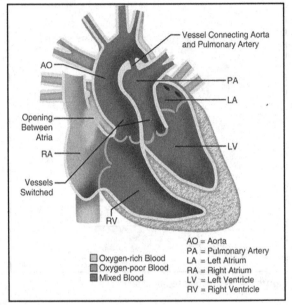

Figure 6-6. Transposition of the great vessels.

require surgery or multiple surgeries to allow the heart to still work despite the problems.

Fun Fact: Medical students and others can remember the five main types of cyanotic congenital heart disease by relying on their fingers and five Ts. Start with a closed fist then:

1. *Hold up one finger—a single great vessel, or Truncus arteriosus*

2. *Hold up two fingers that are crossed—two vessels transposed, or Transposition*

3. *Hold up three fingers—Tricuspid valve atresia*

4. *Hold up four fingers—Tetraology of Fallot, which has four things wrong with the heart*

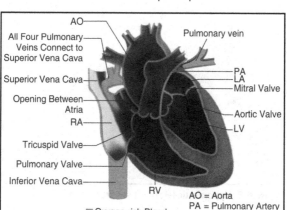

Figure 6-7. Total anomalous venous return.

5. *Hold up all five fingers—Total anomalous pulmonary venous return (five words in the name)*

The cyanotic congenital heart conditions are not the only important anatomic heart defects. One of the most difficult and life-threatening conditions is a hypoplastic left ventricle (Figure 6-8), where the primary pumping ventricle for the heart does not develop normally. This can cause early death, but increasingly can be palliated by a series of heart operations during infancy and childhood. This lesion causes problems because not enough blood is pumped out to the body. However, it is not cyanotic because there is not a problem getting oxygen into the blood through the lungs. Similarly, coarctation of the aorta (Figure 6-9) is a blockage in the major artery leaving the heart and, therefore, it can cause problems getting blood down to the lower half of the body.

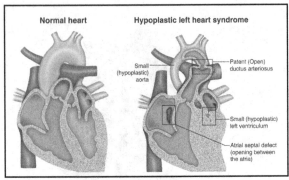

Figure 6-8. Hypoplastic left heart syndrome.

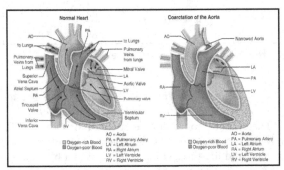

Figure 6-9. Coarctation of the aorta.

In adults, the most common problem in the heart itself is with the arteries that supply blood to the heart muscle, or coronary artery disease. Coronary artery disease can lead to heart attacks because even though the heart has blood flowing through it, the heart muscle depends on a series of small arteries to supply it with the oxygen it needs. Hypertension, stroke, and peripheral artery disease are all common problems of the cardio-vascular system in adults. Peripheral artery disease essentially never happens in children and stroke is rare, but hypertension does occur occasionally for a variety of reasons. Children can acquire heart problems during childhood, but these are uncommon in the United States currently. One of the most common causes of acquired heart problems in children worldwide is rheumatic fever, which leads to problems with the function of one or more of the valves in the heart. Luckily, rheumatic fever is now very rare in the United States.

HYPERTENSION

High blood pressure is not common in children and adolescents compared to adults. However, as children have gotten heavier, hypertension has also become more common. There are also a variety of other causes of hypertension in children (Table 6-1). Similar to determining a normal BMI in children, blood pressure should also be plotted on a chart that displays normal blood pressures for age, height, and sex. However, children should have lower blood pressures than adults, so blood pressures higher than the adult cutoffs are always abnormal.

The first step in measuring blood pressure is to have a child relax in a position where the blood pressure cuff will be at the same level as the heart. If they recently walked into the office, they should rest before having their blood pressure taken. Then, an appropriately sized blood pressure cuff should be selected. There are blood pressure cuffs for premature infants up through adult cuffs originally intended to fit on the thigh of an adult, so you can definitely find a pressure cuff for children of all sizes. The bladder, or balloon part of the cuff that blows up, should cover 80% to 100% of the circumference of the arm, and the cuff should not extend below the bottom of the biceps muscle past the elbow or into the armpit. Definitive blood pressure readings should

Table 6-1
Causes of Hypertension in Children

Infant and Young Children	Older Children and Adolescents
Incorrectly taken blood pressure	Incorrectly taken blood pressure
Renal artery or vein thrombosis or stenosis	Essential (primary) hypertension
Congenital renal malformations	Obesity
Coarctation of the aorta	Renal parenchymal disease or scarring
Neuroblastoma, pheochromocytoma, or other tumors secreting hormones	Neuroblastoma, pheochromocytoma, or other tumors secreting hormones
Patent ductus arteriosus	Renal vascular disease
	Drug ingestions
	Chromosomal syndromes
	Increased intracranial pressure
	Prescribed medications such as steroids

be taken by hand using a stethoscope, but often an automatic blood pressure cuff is used for convenience. Automatic blood pressure cuffs tend to have inaccurate diastolic blood pressure measurements and can be wrong in other ways too, so manual blood pressures should be used to clarify the current status or to make a diagnosis of hypertension. To take the blood pressure, tighten the cuff to a pressure that occludes blood flow to the arm. Then

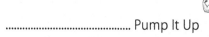

slowly decrease the pressure and listen for the pressure where arterial circulation restarts and the lower number that occurs when the cuff pressure is lower than the pressure in the arteries between pumps of the heart.

Blood pressure higher than the 95th percentile in the population based on age, height, and sex but lower than 5 mm Hg above the 99th percentile is considered stage 1 hypertension if repeatedly found at that level. Stage 2 hypertension is a reading higher than 5 mm Hg above the 99th percentile. *Prehypertension* is a term for children with a blood pressure between the 90th and 95th percentile. Unlike adult patients, where blood pressure cutoffs were developed based on the risk of increased morbidity like stroke or mortality, these exact levels have not been as clearly linked to specific medical problems in children but are thought to increase the risk for stress on the arteries, kidneys, and heart over time and cause problems with those organs. Rarely, children or adolescents will develop onset of hypertension in a short amount of time and have a hypertensive emergency due to the kidneys failing, medication use, or some other reaction. Blood pressures can be so high that children can have strokes, other brain changes, and kidney or heart damage. These hypertensive emergencies are always treated in intensive care units using intravenous medications to slowly lower the blood pressure in a controlled manner.

PAIN IN THE CHEST

As previously stated, heart attacks are rare in children and when they do occur, it is usually because there was a problem with the development of the arteries that supply the heart. However, chest pain is extremely common in children, especially in adolescence. People often worry about the heart, but again chest pain is almost never from

---

Table 6-2
Common Causes of Chest Pain in Children and
Adolescents

- Chest wall pain—from injury, strain, or unclear
  cause
- Asthma
- Lower respiratory tract infection
- Anxiety
- Gastroesophageal reflux
- Precordial catch syndrome

---

the heart in children and adolescents. However, it should
still be evaluated by a physician because there can be
dangerous causes of chest pain that are not due to heart
attacks, such as in Table 6-2.

FAINTING, FALLING-OUT, AND THE DROPSIES IN CHILDREN AND ADOLESCENTS

Fainting, or syncope, is one of the most worrisome
symptoms that develop in children, although like chest
pain, the cause of fainting is usually not dangerous.
However, unlike with chest pain, the resultant fall can
cause injuries from hitting the head or body. Despite
usually benign causes, a physician should evaluate any
children who start having syncope. In very young children, the main cause of fainting that is usually not
dangerous is called a *breath-holding spell*. These spells
can occur from a variety of stimuli. One of the most
common types occurs when infants or young children

cry and cry and cry and essentially run out of air. They have a pause in their breathing, turn a little bluish, and then faint. This can happen after anger, frustration, or injury. Another trigger for these fainting or breath-holding spells can be a painful stimuli, which is similar to adults who become lightheaded and faint. The child does not turn blue and usually does not cry. These children should see their doctor, who usually will provide reassurance in many cases and may treat the child with iron therapy, which appears to treat or reduce the frequency of episodes for many children.

Adolescent fainting is usually due to a combination of cardiac and neural causes that is termed *vasovagal syncope*. In this type of syncope, some stimulus starts a neural reflex that causes stimulation of the vagal nerve and resultant hypotension, a slow heart rate, and dilation of the peripheral vasculature. Triggers of this experience can be emotional stress, such as seeing or hearing something shocking, blood draws, or other painful stimuli. In addition, dehydration, prolonged standing, or heat exposure and exertion can simulate this physiology and cause similar symptoms. Not feeling good, pallor, nausea, and sweating, which are all controlled by the same vagal part of the nervous system, often precede this type of fainting. The person can then either fall or slump into a seated or lying position and become unconscious. Sometimes there can be a slight amount of muscle twitching, causing people to think it is a seizure, but in reality, it is not a seizure. Usually, people wake up relatively quickly, but often are severely fatigued and slowed for hours after it happens. Again, unless the episode was obviously this type, it is reasonable to seek medical evaluation because there are causes of syncope that are signs of underlying medical problems. Table 6-3 lists some of the more worrisome signs associated with syncope that definitely warrant medical evaluation.

Table 6-3
Worrisome Types of Fainting

- During exercising or running (less worrisome if after exercise when resting)
- Family history of unexplained or cardiac death
- Accompanied by exertional chest pain
- Palpitations or rapid or irregular heartbeat before the event
- After a loud sound
- Focal neurologic deficits when they wake up
- Unclear speech or "spinning of room" when wake up
- Syncope without any preceding symptoms

Chapter 7

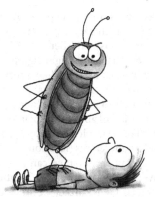

Bugs Galore
and More
(Gastroenterology)

"My stomach hurts." How many times has this statement been heard coming out of a child's mouth? Hopefully that is all that is coming out of the mouth. Gastrointestinal complaints are common among children, and this chapter will give an overview about abdominal pain and poop—probably more than you ever wanted to know.

Steiner MJ, Kimple KS. *The Little Book of Pediatrics: Infants to Teens and Everything in Between* (pp 91-104).
© 2016 Taylor & Francis Group.

STARTS WITH A STORY

Abdominal pain is common but its cause is not always easily diagnosed, which can make parents and pediatric providers a little uneasy and perhaps a bit queasy. The patient's history is critical in figuring out what is going on with abdominal pain (seems like a recurring theme). It can be easier to think of abdominal pain as acute versus chronic or recurrent to narrow the long list of causes. In addition, the location of abdominal pain (or lack thereof) can be helpful. For example, mid-upper abdominal pain can be caused by pancreatitis (location of the pancreas) or pain of the right upper abdomen can be caused by right lower lung, liver, or biliary problems (location of the liver and biliary tract). Generalized, poorly described pain can be typical of functional abdominal pain of childhood (more on this later). Any associated symptoms (ie, diarrhea or vomiting—or both in those lucky individuals) can also be insightful, as well as "alarm findings," or signs and symptoms that make a medical cause more likely. Even if a provider cannot find an exact etiology, ruling out the serious and life-threatening causes of abdominal pain is the first step.

RUNNING OFF THE TRACT

Acute abdominal pain has a variety of causes and can be different depending on the age and gender of the child. Table 7-1 includes many of these causes, in no particular order. A commonly feared cause is appendicitis, which is typically seen in a child older than 2 years. Symptoms can vary, especially in younger children, but the classic presentation is right lower quadrant abdominal pain (may start as more generalized pain around belly button and then move down and localize to the right

Table 7-1
Causes of Acute Abdominal Pain in Children

- Abdominal migraine
- Adhesions (leads to intestinal obstruction)
- Appendicitis
- Necrotizing enterocolitis
- Volvulus
- Milk protein allergy
- Testicular torsion
- Foreign body ingestion
- Hemolytic uremic syndrome
- Hirschsprung's disease/enterocolitis
- Incarcerated hernia
- Intussusception
- Trauma
- Gastroenteritis
- Viral illness
- Hepatitis
- Vaso-occlusive crisis in sickle cell disease
- Toxin/poisoning (ie, lead)
- Tumor
- Urinary tract infection
- Spontaneous bacterial peritonitis (complication of nephrotic syndrome or ascites)
- Pharyngitis (ie, strep)
- Constipation
- Henoch–Schönlein purpura
- Intra-abdominal abscess
- Meckel's diverticulum
- Ovarian torsion
- Pneumonia
- Diabetic ketoacidosis
- Myocarditis/pericarditis

(continued)

Table 7-1
Causes of Acute Abdominal Pain in Children
(continued)

- Peptic ulcer disease/perforated ulcer
- Cholecystitis
- Familial Mediterranean fever
- Hyperimmunoglobulin D syndrome
- Inflammatory bowel disease
- Ruptured ovarian cyst
- Pancreatitis
- Urolithiasis (kidney stones)
- Ectopic pregnancy
- Mesenteric lymphadenitis
- Acute porphyria

lower quadrant), nausea, vomiting, and a low-grade fever in a child who does not want to eat (asking the child if he or she is hungry can be a key question…but do not give food just in case surgery is needed). The main treatment for appendicitis is surgical removal. We do not need our appendix anyway.

Another serious cause of acute abdominal pain is intussusception, which is a common cause of obstruction that occurs when the bowel telescopes into itself and is usually seen between age 3 months and 6 years. If not treated, it can cause loss of blood flow to the bowel, bowel perforation, or even death, although occasionally the telescoping can be intermittent or even resolve on its own. The usual presentation in a child is sudden onset of abdominal pain and frequent attacks of pain where the child typically pulls the legs up and cries. Vomiting is also common. There may be a tender "sausage-like" mass when examining the abdomen, but this is not always present. If not treated promptly, the child may become lethargic and develop bloody, mucous-like stools (some have been known to compare it to "currant jelly"). X-rays of the abdomen may reveal abnormalities but may be normal, so it is also important to check stool for blood. If intussusception is suspected, then a contrast or air enema can diagnose and fix the problem at the same time. However, occasionally, the contrast or air enema is not successful and the child will have to undergo surgery.

Acute abdominal pain can also be caused by viral or bacterial gastroenteritis, or the "the stomach bug" as some like to call it. The "bug" is most commonly a virus, but bacterial causes are important to consider from exposures such as animals (those lovely petting zoos) or undercooked or contaminated food. Parasitic infections are also possible, but these infections usually follow an exposure, such as traveling abroad or drinking contaminated water (ie, *Giardia*) and if not recognized, can be a cause of chronic abdominal pain. Rotavirus used to be the most common etiology of diarrheal illness in children until the rotavirus vaccine was introduced in 2006.

In gastroenteritis, abdominal pain is frequently accompanied by vomiting and then diarrhea and sometimes fever. Bacterial gastroenteritis can cause bloody diarrhea, and certain bacterial infections can lead to later complications (such as kidney failure from hemolytic uremic syndrome). Treatment for viral gastroenteritis is patience and time, but it is important to stay hydrated and young children may require intravenous fluids in the hospital for dehydration in severe cases. Small and frequent amounts of clear fluids by mouth work well for oral rehydration, which is the best way to stay hydrated in cases that are not as severe. For bacterial gastroenteritis, antibiotics are occasionally necessary in some infections to shorten their duration or prevent complications but not always. Antibiotics are also used in children with compromised immune systems or in the case of *Clostridium difficile* infection. *C difficile* infection can cause abdominal pain, diarrhea, fever, or even abdominal distension and is usually seen following antibiotic use.

Fun Fact: Toddlers between ages 1 and 3 years may develop intermittently loose stools (called "toddler's diarrhea"), which is usually caused by lots of sugary beverages or juice—cutting down on these will help firm things up.

Acute abdominal pain may not always be from the gastrointestinal tract, and it is important to broaden one's thinking. For example, a urinary tract infection, kidney stones, or even pneumonia in the lower lobes of the lungs can cause abdominal pain. Girls may present with abdominal pain from problems with the reproductive system, such as ovulation, an ovarian cyst, an ectopic pregnancy, or even chlamydia. Boys may also have abdominal pain from testicular torsion, so a complete evaluation is warranted.

PERSISTENT BUGGERS

Abdominal pain that lingers or comes back repeatedly is considered chronic or recurrent abdominal pain, and many of the potential etiologies are included in Table 7-2. Children with chronic or recurrent abdominal pain more commonly have a "functional" disorder, or a pattern of symptoms and pain not related to an organic problem, rather than a serious medical condition. Organic causes of abdominal pain are more likely in children with so-called "alarm findings," and these children should have additional work-up. These findings include weight loss, swallowing problems, significant vomiting (especially bilious), severe or chronic diarrhea, night awakenings from symptoms, unexplained fever, urinary symptoms, back pain, family history of inflammatory bowel disease or celiac disease, bloody diarrhea, melena (black, tarry stools), or skin changes/rashes. In addition, those children with localized abdominal tenderness, oral

Table 7-2
Causes of Chronic or Recurrent Abdominal Pain in Children

- Functional abdominal pain
- Functional dyspepsia
- Irritable bowel syndrome
- Abdominal migraine
- Peptic disorders
- Reflux esophagitis
- Gastritis
- Gastric or duodenal ulcers
- *Helicobacter pylori* infection
- Carbohydrate malabsorption (ie, lactose intolerance)
- Celiac disease
- Constipation/functional constipation
- Dysmenorrhea
- Gastroesophageal reflux
- Esophagitis
- Eosinophilic disorders (esophagitis, gastritis)
- Excess fructose or sorbitol ingestion
- Musculoskeletal pain
- Parasitic infection (ie, *Giardia*)
- Endometriosis
- Inflammatory bowel disease (Crohn's disease or ulcerative colitis)
- Pelvic inflammatory disease
- Urinary tract infection
- Bezoar
- Burkitt lymphoma
- Recurrent intussusception
- Chronic hepatitis
- Chronic pancreatitis

(continued)

Table 7-2
Causes of Chronic or Recurrent Abdominal Pain in Children (continued)

- Familial Mediterranean fever
- Foreign body
- Gallstones, choledochal cyst, chronic cholecystitis
- Heavy metal poisoning (ie, lead)
- Hereditary angioedema
- Imperforate hymen with hematocolpos (menstrual blood fills vagina)
- Malrotation
- Hernia (inguinal or abdominal wall)
- Mesenteric ischemia
- Nephrolithiasis
- Psoas abscess
- Ureteropelvic junction obstruction
- Vasculitis (ie, Henoch–Schönlein purpura)
- Acute intermittent porphyria

---

ulcers, changes in growth, arthritis, an enlarged liver or spleen, tenderness on the back over the kidneys, abnormalities around the anus (eg, tags, fissures), or blood in the stool are also more likely to have an organic reason for abdominal pain.

The most common cause of chronic abdominal pain in children and adolescents is functional abdominal pain. In addition to functional abdominal pain of childhood, this group of disorders includes functional dyspepsia, irritable bowel syndrome, and abdominal migraines. The pain is thought to be related to multiple factors of the gastrointestinal tract and nervous system with increased perception of pain or stretching. It can be diagnosed in children who have abdominal pain at least once per week for more than 2 months and no evidence of an organic problem, including no alarm findings (discussed previously), negative testing for occult blood in stool, and a normal physical examination. The Rome criteria is a tool providers use to make a clinical diagnosis. Management can be a challenge, with a goal of maintaining day-to-day functioning, although psychological support or counseling has been shown to help many children. In most children, abdominal pain resolves with time. However, a child with functional abdominal pain could present with an organic problem as well, so beware.

Constipation is another common cause of chronic or recurrent abdominal pain that can also cause acute abdominal pain. Constipated children have infrequent stools, hard stools, and difficulty passing stools. There is wide variation in what is normal frequency for stooling, so a child with infrequent soft stools does not have constipation. For the most part, constipation in children is considered functional constipation and is not caused by an organic process. If not treated, constipation can be a challenge because the child will further withhold stool because of hard, large stools, resulting in distension and decreased sensation and a poorly functioning stooling reflex. This can result in encopresis, or leakage of watery fecal material around impacted hard stool, which some may even mistake for diarrhea…a vicious cycle.

Organic causes of constipation are infrequent but should not be ruled out, especially in an infant. For example, a newborn who does not stool may have Hirschsprung's disease/enterocolitis, where the nerves are not present at the final part of the colon, resulting in retained stool, a distended abdomen, and a sick infant. Anatomic problems (eg, anal stenosis), neurologic problems (eg, spina bifida), hormonal problems (eg, hypothyroidism), intestinal problems (eg, celiac disease), or medications can all cause constipation. Children with a fever, vomiting, poor feeding, bloody diarrhea, trouble

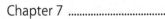

gaining weight, no stool in a tight rectum, or an abscess around the rectum should be evaluated further for possible organic causes. Treatment is aimed at correcting an organic problem if one exists or close management with medications, including a "cleanout" if fecal impaction is present, dietary changes, and behavioral education. Constipation can be a challenge to treat, adding a headache to the bellyache for some.

Chronic abdominal pain with or without chronic diarrhea can be caused by inflammation of the bowel due to *celiac disease* or *IBD*. Celiac disease is an autoimmune disease where the gluten protein in wheat stimulates the inflammation. IBD is a term used for *Crohn's disease* and *ulcerative colitis*, which are problems of chronic inflammation of the intestines. Crohn's disease can affect any area of the digestive tract (from mouth to anus), whereas ulcerative colitis involves the colon, as the name implies. This distinction is not always clear cut and the two can overlap or even be called *indeterminate colitis* if a child is not following all of the rules. The cause is not exactly known, although it is thought to be a combination of genetic predisposition and influences from the environment. Although IBD can be seen in younger children, it more commonly affects adolescents and can present with abdominal pain, weight loss, diarrhea, anemia, or even symptoms outside of the gut. Ulcerative colitis presents more with bloody diarrhea and occasionally a severe urge to go to the bathroom, whereas Crohn's disease may present more with weight loss, poor growth, or even delayed sexual development. These children will need endoscopy (using a camera from above or below to look at the inside of the bowel and take biopsies). Visuals can also be obtained with new technology, such as tiny cameras that are swallowed, to get to hard-to-reach places.

IN RETROGRADE

If all of that complaining about abdominal pain is coming out of the mouth along with vomiting, hope there is a toilet or trashcan nearby. Vomiting can be a symptom caused by many disorders and may be present alone or accompanied by other symptoms. Although vomiting can be due to common causes such as gastroenteritis, it can also be a sign of serious illnesses, such as diabetic ketoacidosis, metabolic problems (otherwise known as inborn errors of metabolism), or even a brain tumor, so it is important to take a good history. If you thought you had enough hearing about the consistency and color of stool, now you can inquire about the details of emesis. Vomiting can be bilious (bright green color) or non-bilious. Bilious vomiting is more concerning because this can be a sign of intestinal obstruction since things will come back up the mouth if there is nowhere to go. Volvulus is a life-threatening cause of bilious vomiting and occurs when the bowel twists on itself, usually as a result of the bowel being malrotated from not finalizing its position during fetal development. The most common cause of serious non-bilious vomiting in infants (not to be confused with regurgitation or reflux present in all infants) is pyloric stenosis, causing obstruction of the stomach outlet, and surgical intervention is required. Vomiting in this case usually starts around age 3 to 4 weeks but can occur up to age 5 months.

Since we are on the subject of things coming back up the digestive tract, let's talk about a common esophageal problem in children: gastroesophageal reflux (or gastroesophageal reflux disease [GERD], if it is really a problem). In infants, reflux or regurgitation is universal, with "spit up" happening all over the place. This usually starts in the first couple months of life and can get worse up to about age 4 months. Overfeeding can contribute

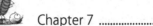

to or worsen reflux. Infants can occasionally choke or cough and some seem more bothered by it whereas others have no associated symptoms. In severe cases, an infant may not be able to gain weight appropriately or may develop an aversion to feeding. Older children and adolescents may not spit up, but may complain of abdominal and chest pain due to reflux or even chronic cough. Treatment options for GERD in infants include controlling the volume and speed of feedings, thickening milk with rice cereal, and, if infants are not gaining weight, changing to a different formula due to a possible milk protein allergy. Medications or antacids are used in infants and children in the short-term to reduce irritation and the acidity of what comes up but they do not stop anything from coming up. In severe, intractable cases, a surgical procedure called a *Nissen fundoplication* can be considered.

RED IS THE NEW BLACK

Blood in a child's stool can be very concerning but is not always cause for concern. Of course, providers should rule out serious causes, but it could be swallowed maternal blood (from birth or nipple bleeding) in infants or a tear around the rectum, known as an anal fissure. An anal fissure is the most common cause of blood in the stool of young children. The amount, color, and pattern of bleeding are always good to ask. For example, a little bit of bright red blood around the stool may be from stool passing by an anal fissure, whereas a significant amount of blood in the toilet bowl water warrants further investigation. Dark or black stools can suggest upper gastrointestinal bleeding from stomach or peptic ulcers. You can think of it as having a longer trip and taking all day to get there, so it is dark by the time it arrives. Stool can also be red from certain food or drinks, so it is important to confirm suspected bleeding with a test for occult blood on a stool sample.

In infants, a relatively common cause of red blood in the stool (known as hematochezia) is milk protein allergy. Symptoms of milk protein allergy can range from skin problems (such as atopic dermatitis) to blood in the stool, GERD, constipation, or failure to thrive/ poor weight gain. If a child has blood in the stool, significant symptoms, or is not gaining weight, treatment options are to change from a cow's milk–based formula to a hydrolyzed or amino acid–based formula or for the breastfeeding mother to avoid all milk products. Soy formula is not a good substitute because many children with a milk protein allergy will also react to soy.

LAMENTING LIVERS

Although problems can arise in any organ in the abdomen, we will briefly mention liver problems, specifically hepatitis. People often use the term *hepatitis* to refer to a specific group of viral infections, but in reality hepatitis solely means inflammation of the liver and can have a variety of causes, including a toxic ingestion (including alcohol), various viral infections, medication side effects, autoimmune illness, and fat deposition in the liver. The specific hepatitis viruses that are most frequently discussed are hepatitis A, B, and C. Hepatitis A is passed through food-borne infections and causes liver inflammation and associated jaundice and vomiting. People almost universally recover and it does not cause chronic liver disease. Hepatitis B is passed sexually through blood and other body fluids or through maternal transmission to the infant and can cause chronic liver disease. Hepatitis C is passed through perinatal transmission or blood, such as with sharing needles, although passing in other body fluids is also possible. Many adults with hepatitis C have no symptoms, so some groups now recommend screening for this infection. Others can develop chronic liver disease and die from hepatitis C. Despite the serious nature of chronic hepatitis, most people who develop acute inflammation of the liver from various causes have mild disease that resolves without any long-term problems.

HELLO YELLOW

Jaundice, or yellowing of the skin, can be a sign of problems with the liver or biliary tract but can also be common in newborns. Bilirubin is responsible for the yellow color and is measured in the blood as direct or indirect. A high indirect bilirubin in a newborn, especially one born prematurely, is typical of neonatal hyperbilirubinemia or neonatal jaundice. This is due to an immature liver and trouble removing bilirubin from the body effectively, so it builds up. Jaundice can be seen more commonly with breastfeeding infants, especially because the amount of milk is related to enterohepatic circulation of bilirubin and it can take a little longer for breastmilk to come in after birth. This is different from breastmilk jaundice, which is benign and starts about 1 to 2 weeks after birth and can occur up to 6 weeks after a healthy full-term birth. Occasionally, an infant has an indirect bilirubin level that is too high and requires treatment to prevent complications, such as damage to the brain (kernicterus). Phototherapy, or light therapy, is used to help break the bilirubin down so the body can get rid of it.

Chapter 8

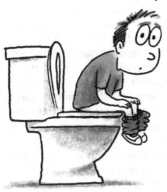

To Pee or Not to Pee (Renal/Genitourinary)

CARE OF GENITALIA IN NEWBORNS AND YOUNG CHILDREN

The genitalia of little boys and girls generally needs cleaning, care, and attention that is similar to other parts of the body. Most newborns do not need frequent baths,

Steiner MJ, Kimple KS. *The Little Book of Pediatrics: Infants to Teens and Everything in Between* (pp 105-119).
© 2016 Taylor & Francis Group.

but washing children off with water, a very gentle soap, and a washcloth for bath time can create fun, quality time for parents and infants.

Parents should know that newborn girls often have vaginal discharge that is sometimes bloody, which is related to the removal of maternal hormones and establishment of their own hormonal axis. Newborns can also have some pinkish granules in their urine. These urate crystals are a normal and common finding in newborns. To keep the genitalia of female infants clean, soaking in a bath and using a gentle soap or use of a washcloth on the outside of the labia is fine.

Little boys are born with an intact penis that includes a foreskin that covers the entire glans. Most boys have a urethra that opens on the tip of the penis, but this opening can be located away from the tip of the penis, which is called *hypospadias* (below the tip or underside of penis) or *epispadias* (above the tip or the upper aspect of penis). If one of these conditions is noticed, a urology specialist should evaluate the newborn. Infants who are not circumcised will not be able to have the skin of the penis pulled back to expose the glans. Caregivers should not attempt to do this because it is painful and the skin can get stuck in that position. As boys grow and their penises grow, the foreskin will gradually be able to be retracted over the glans, with the majority able to do this by age 2 or 3 years. As the newborns grow, parents can gently push back the skin and clean with warm water and a washcloth, but again, the skin should not be forced back.

CIRCUMCISION OR NO CIRCUMCISION

The current recommendations on circumcision are that overall there are medical benefits to circumcision, but it remains a family decision that is influenced by parental preferences and cultural beliefs. In many states, public insurance does not currently pay for circumcision, although some recent analyses of the cost and long-term benefits suggest that circumcision may be cost saving for insurance companies.[1] The primary benefits of circumcision are that it reduces the risk of urinary tract infections (UTIs) in the first year of life and reduces the risk of sexually transmitted infections later in life. The primary risk of circumcision that is concretely known is a risk of bleeding during and immediately after the procedure. For families that choose not to circumcise, it may be a cultural tradition that it is not done, parents may choose to avoid procedures that are not necessary, or some parents may be concerned that circumcision changes penile sensation later in life.

There are three commonly accepted ways to perform neonatal infant circumcision. The first uses a Gomco clamp, and the foreskin is cut off immediately after a small thimble-like object is fitted over the glans, or head of the penis. The second uses a Mogen clamp, and the foreskin is pulled forward and incised across the skin. Finally, a Plasti-bell circumcision places a plastic thimble-like device over the glans, the foreskin is pulled over the thimble, and a tight tie is put around the foreskin so that the foreskin dies and falls off over the subsequent week.

Regardless of the type of circumcision, it is the current standard of practice to use a local anesthetic, as well as systemic soothing and pain relief, often using a pacifier with sugar on it and possibly acetaminophen. Infant circumcision is typically done at the end of the first day of life through age 1 to 2 weeks in the United States. If an indication for circumcision occurs after age 2 to 3 months, then in the United States the circumcision is generally done in the operating room or under sedation. After a child is circumcised, it will take 1 week or more for the skin to fully heal. Vaseline should be applied to the glans twice daily until the skin has fully healed and the glans no longer appears irritated. Thereafter, the skin left on the penile shaft should gently be pulled back when the baby is given a bath and the glans should be cleaned with water.

URINARY TRACT INFECTIONS: FEVER, BURNING, AND PAIN...OH MY

Children and young adults of any age can get UTIs. In infants and young children, a UTI is an important cause of fever and morbidity and can be a presenting sign of an anatomic problem in the urinary tract system. Approximately 1% of boys and 3% of girls are diagnosed with a UTI before puberty and this is the most common serious bacterial infection in infants.[2] Approximately 70% of infants with a UTI and fever also have a kidney infection and approximately 5% of infants with a UTI also have the bacteria cultured from their bloodstream, so these infections can definitely be serious.[3] A common anatomic problem associated with UTIs is something called *vesicoureteral reflux* (VUR). For children with VUR, urine moves from the kidney to the ureter to the bladder but can also reflux back up into the ureter or, in severe cases, back up into the kidney. This urine that washes back and forth has an increased risk for infection, and kidney infections can cause kidney scarring and damage. Another anatomic problem in male infants associated with UTIs and even more serious kidney problems is posterior urethral valves. These valves are the result of abnormal development in utero and can block the bladder of male infants from emptying. This causes problems due to pressure backing up into the bladder and kidney, but also often presents by male infants getting a UTI because the urine is not emptying normally.

Infants with UTIs often present with a fever and no other known symptoms, and older children may present with burning or pain during urination; in these cases, the urine itself can be tested for a UTI. In infants, urine can be collected using a bag adhered to the perineum; however, if a culture to grow bacteria is necessary, then a small catheter is usually introduced into the urethra to obtain urine so the sample is not contaminated from the skin around the urethra. In older children, the urine can be collected from the middle of a stream while the child is urinating. A urinalysis is the first test most clinicians order. This is completed by using a strip of paper with various areas containing different reagents that react to certain colors based on the urine components. This can be used to examine various components of the urine and is summarized in Table 8-1.

After a urinalysis is done, clinicians or laboratory technicians can look at the urine under a microscope, allowing people to directly see bacteria and white blood cells. However, it is also possible to see red blood cells, other cells from the kidney or bladder, crystals in the urine, clumpings of cells from injured kidneys, and a large amount of other interesting and important information about the urinary tract. Finally, a UTI is confirmed by actually growing the bacteria in a culture medium. It usually takes at least 18 to 24 hours to identify the bacteria grown from the urine, so occasionally treatment starts before this final answer is definitively known. UTIs in infants older than age 1 to 2 months and children can be treated with oral antibiotics, assuming the child is not vomiting up the medication. Infants younger than that are usually admitted to the hospital and often have had other blood or spinal fluid tests done to evaluate fevers before the urine is confirmed as the source.

After toilet training but before puberty, it is somewhat unusual for children to have UTIs unless they have previously had infections. It definitely can happen, and sometimes is associated with constipation or some other issue that creates an environment in which bacteria have

Table 8-1
Components of Many Urinalysis Dip Sticks

Specific gravity	Measures how concentrated the urine is based on weight of the urine compared to water.
pH	Urine is used by the body to maintain a normal acidity in the body. The pH of urine can vary based on things happening in the body.
Blood	Detects heme or iron in the urine that usually is from blood in the urine. There are other things that contain iron and can come out in the urine like some muscle proteins.
Leukocyte esterase	Detects an enzyme that is released by white blood cells or infection-fighting cells when they are in the urine. It almost always tests positively if a urine infection is present.
Nitrite	Detects nitrite, which is converted from nitrate by the most common bacteria that cause urinary tract infections. If this is positive, children usually do have a urinary tract infection.

(continued)

Table 8-1
Components of Many Urinalysis Dip Sticks (continued)

Protein	Detects albumin in the urine, which is a large protein that is commonly leaked in various types of kidney disease.
Glucose	Detects the presence of glucose in the urine. Glucose only goes into the urine when the serum/blood glucose is over approximately 180 or 200 mg/dL. There are some rare kidney conditions that leak glucose at lower serum glucose levels.
Ketones	Detects ketones, which are created by the body when fat is used as a fuel. The presence of large amount of ketones suggests fasting or not eating carbohydrates recently or complications of diabetes.

an easier time establishing an infection in the bladder. Children who have early infections often can continue having infections when school-aged, particularly if they have VUR or another anatomic variant that predisposes them to UTIs. When adolescents begin having UTIs as a new problem, it is often associated with the onset of sexual activity. The term for this used to be *honeymoon cystitis,* but it does not have to have occurred on the honeymoon anymore. Adolescent girls or boys with urinary symptoms like burning, frequent urination but not feeling like they completely emptied their bladder, or urgency to go quickly should have a urinalysis performed and can be empirically treated for a bacterial UTI while waiting for the bacterial culture. However, if the culture results were negative or if girls have other vaginal symptoms, like discharge or lower abdominal pain, then they need to be evaluated for other causes of pain and dysuria that do not grow bacteria on standard culture plates, such as sexually transmitted infections.

SEXUALLY TRANSMITTED INFECTIONS

Sexually transmitted genital infections are remarkably common. The average age of first intercourse in US females is 16 years, and 25% of adolescents aged 14 to 19 years have a sexually transmitted infection.[4] Approximately 20% have been exposed to human papillomavirus (HPV), which causes cervical and vaginal cancer, 5% have chlamydia, 3% have trichomonas, and 2% have gonorrhea or herpes.[5] The percentage of girls with some type of sexually transmitted infection increases to 40% if you only include girls who acknowledge sexual activity.[5] Gonorrhea and chlamydia can lead to acute pelvic inflammatory disease (PID) over time and to permanent infertility. Herpes causes painful recurrent ulcers, and HPV can cause cancer and warts.

Due to the high prevalence, potential for asymptomatic carrier states, and long-term problems associated with these infections, providers should screen sexually active teenagers for chlamydia and gonorrhea annually. These infections can now be tested for using either urinary tests or vaginal self-swabs. Testing for cervical dysplasia and HPV is now delayed until age 21 years; however, early vaccination can prevent the more virulent species of HPV. In addition, HIV testing is now recommended for all adolescents annually and syphilis serologic testing can be performed in high-risk areas. If adolescents present with genital symptoms, they should not only be screened as above, but also be examined for bacterial vaginosis and trichomoniasis. If clinical examination is concerning for PID in female adolescents or purulent cervicitis without upper genital tract symptoms, then empiric antibiotic therapy is indicated.

CONTRACEPTION

Discussions about contraception and its use in adolescents can be a controversial area in pediatric practice. In many states, adolescents can consent for treatment around sexual health without parental involvement. Although the payment systems for this confidential care can be complicated, the intent of the laws in those states is clear—adolescents should be able to have some independent control over their reproductive systems when under the care of a health care provider.

The primary goal of contraception is to prevent unintended pregnancy from sexual encounters. In addition, some contraceptive options decrease the risk of sexually transmitted infections, and others improve acne, menstrual regularity, and menstrual discomfort. However, contraception can have risks, particularly when it involves systemic hormonal therapy; however, the risks of all contraception are lower than the medical risk associated with pregnancy.

There are a variety of options for contraception, although the majority continues to be dependent on young women bearing the ultimate responsibility. Table 8-2 includes the currently available options in the United States, with associated comments about each method. We have not included permanent sterilization, such as tubal ligation or vasectomy, because these would only be used for adolescent patients in extreme, unique situations. One note about recent developments in contraceptive options is that long-acting reversible contraception is now considered a first-line option for adolescent patients. Previous concern about the long-term impact or acute complications related to sexually transmitted infections are clearly outweighed by the dramatically improved real-world efficacy of these methods to prevent pregnancy for adolescents who are often unable to consistently use other methods. Examples of long-acting, reversible contraception available in the United States include three different intrauterine devices and a subcutaneous progesterone implant. Medical providers and adolescents should begin using these as a primary option for prevention of pregnancy.

PROTEINURIA AND HEMATURIA

Proteinuria is when a significant amount of protein, particularly a protein called albumin, is detectable in the urine. Hematuria is when blood is notable in the urine. Protein can occur in large or trace amounts, occur after standing all day, occur intermittently, or be constant. Similarly, hematuria can be microscopic only or not visible, intermittent, and from either the lower urinary tract or from the upper tract and kidney. Children with persistent blood or protein in the urine need to have a

Table 8-2
Contraceptive Options for Adolescents in the United States (Ordered Approximately From Least to Most Effective)

Method	Male or Female Use	Comments
Spermicide	F	Ineffective with a 28% failure rate in a year of regular intercourse.[6]
Timing method	M/F	Adolescent ovulatory irregularities and impulsivity make this method even more ineffective than for adults.
Withdrawal	M/F	Pre-ejaculatory emissions can include sperm and decreased sexual experience among adolescents make this method highly ineffective.
Condom	M	Female condoms have not been marketed widely in the United States. Condoms are beneficial in preventing sexually transmitted infections.
Sponge	F	Relatively effective. Female insertion prior to intercourse. Not widely used.

(continued)

Table 8-2

Contraceptive Options for Adolescents in the United States (Ordered Approximately From Least to Most Effective) (continued)

Method	Male or Female Use	Comments
Diaphragm	F	Must be correctly inserted to cover cervix at each sexual encounter.
Contraceptive ring	F	Inserted and left in place for 3 weeks per month. Some systemic estrogen effects.
Patch	F	Changed weekly. Similar to oral combined contraceptives with slightly increased clotting risk due to higher estrogen dose.
Oral contraceptives	F	A longer standing form of contraception. Required to take a medication consistently and every day.
Injectable progesterone	F	Highly effective, a shot is administered every 3 months. Generally administered in a medical office so requires an office visit every 3 months.

(continued)

Table 8-2
Contraceptive Options for Adolescents in the United States (Ordered Approximately From Least to Most Effective) (continued)

Method	Male or Female Use	Comments
Intrauterine device	F	Highly effective. Risk of PID if infection currently occurring at insertion. Lasts between 5 and 10 years.
Progesterone implant	F	Highly effective. Technically lasts 3 years but likely can last longer.
Post-coital Contraception: Less Effective than Highly Effective Methods		
Morning-after pill	F	A variety of combinations available, taken the sooner after coitus the more effective. Available over the counter after a certain age.

complete evaluation by a physician because this some-times suggests an injury to or problem with the kidneys that can be very serious.

The most common cause of abnormal amounts of protein in the urine for children is due to something called *minimal change disease*. This problem can usually be effectively treated but can be dangerous if not recog-nized and treated aggressively. Orthostatic proteinuria is a less worrisome cause of protein in the urine and is relatively common in adolescents. In this syndrome, the kidney leaks a minor amount of protein during the day while the adolescent is standing and exercising, but if you check the urine after lying down all night, the protein has cleared from the urine.

Blood can appear in the urine during UTIs, during menses, or occasionally during trauma. However, these lower genital tract causes of bleeding are generally less worrisome than causes where the kidneys are leaking red blood cells. Blood from the kidneys is a sign that the glomeruli, or the part of the kidney that filters the blood, are not working correctly. The most common cause of this glomerular dysfunction in children, or glomerulo-nephritis, is called *post-streptococcal glomerulonephritis*. In this syndrome, the infection causes an immune-based reaction that injures the kidney. Children often notice dark brown urine from the large amount of blood pres-ent, swelling, and elevated blood pressure. This problem is usually self-limiting, but supportive hospital care is sometimes needed when the diagnosis is unclear or if blood pressure is dangerously elevated. There are a large number of other glomerular diseases that cause blood in the urine, but assessment and treatment of those can become complicated. Of note, small amounts of blood that are not visible but only detected on a urinalysis test in children are rarely dangerous and often need little work-up or evaluation.

REFERENCES

1. Kacker S, Frick K, Gaydos C, Tobian A. Costs and effectiveness of neonatal male circumcision. *Arch Pediatr Adolesc Med.* 2012;166(10):910.

2. Coplen D. Urinary tract infection: clinical practice guideline for the diagnosis and management of the initial uti in febrile infants and children 2 to 24 months. *Yearbook of Urology.* 2012;2012:236-237.

3. Hoberman A, Charron M, Hickey R, Baskin M, Kearney D, Wald E. Imaging studies after a first febrile urinary tract infection in young children. *N Engl J Med.* 2003;348(3):195-202.

4. Martinez G, Copen CE, Abma JC. Teenagers in the united states: sexual activity, contraceptive use, and childbearing, 2006–2010 national survey of family growth. *Vital Health Stat 23.* 2011;31:1-35.

5. Forhan S, Gottlieb S, Sternberg M et al. Prevalence of sexually transmitted infections among female adolescents aged 14 to 19 in the united states. *Pediatrics.* 2009;124(6):1505-1512.

6. Centers for Disease Control and Prevention. Effectiveness of Family Planning Methods. 2015. Available at: http://www.cdc.gov/reproductivehealth/UnintendedPregnancy/PDF/Contraceptive_methods_508.pdf. Accessed August 25, 2015.

Chapter 9

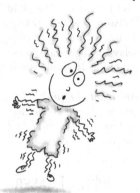

Shake, Ache,
Rattle, and Roll
(Neurology)

It's All in Your Head

The brain is an amazing organ, but it can really leave your head spinning trying to navigate the world of neurology. Neurologic problems in childhood vary from common headaches to rare, devastating disorders of the

Steiner MJ, Kimple KS. *The Little Book of Pediatrics: Infants to Teens and Everything in Between* (pp 121-138).

brain. Because we cannot always know what is going on in that head, it is important to get a good, complete history from the family and the child if possible. The developmental history is especially important in children because their brains are rapidly changing and advancing and because delays or regression in development can be a clue that something is going on within the nervous system.

Fun Fact: An infant's brain doubles in size in the first year of life, forming neuron connections at an incredibly fast rate. Around age 2 or 3 years, the brain has twice as many neuron connections as an adult.

MIND ERASER

An unfortunate condition in children who have over-all brain dysfunction is called *encephalopathy* (generally meaning disease of the brain). Encephalopathy has many causes, including different kinds of infections, toxins, metabolic disorders, lack of oxygen to the brain, and head injury and can be permanent or progressive. One type is static encephalopathy, which is a more general term for unchanging, or static, brain damage. Cerebral palsy is an example of static encephalopathy and is the most common physical disability in children. Cerebral palsy occurs from problems in early brain development, leading to motor difficulties and often accompanied by other problems. It can be a result of different etiologies, including infections, genetic or metabolic problems, and lack of oxygen to the brain, which lead to symptoms of varying severity. In most cases, something happens before birth that causes abnormal brain development, with few experiencing an event after birth. Others may have a congenital problem that affects brain development. Cerebral palsy occurs more often in premature infants (especially those weighing less than 1 kg at birth), given the risk of bleeding into the brain (intracerebral hemorrhage) and periventricular leukomalacia (damage to the white matter of the brain). Although symptoms vary, children with cerebral palsy typically have muscle weakness, poor motor control, and spasticity (or excessive muscle tightening and stiffness). In addition, they may have negative effects on other parts of their brain, including cognitive impairment, seizures, learning disabilities, behavioral problems, or vision, hearing, or speech problems. However, many children with cerebral palsy have totally normal cognitive ability.

Classically, cerebral palsy is described in four different categories depending on the presentation (Table 9-1). These include spastic hemiplegia (increased tone in half of the body), spastic diplegia (increased tone in both legs), spastic quadriplegia (increased tone in arms and legs, with legs worse than arms), and extrapyramidal or athetoid (increased tone in arms, legs and movement problems) cerebral palsy. Spasticity refers to the muscles having increased tone, or hypertonicity. For example, a child with spastic diplegia may present with delayed walking and walking on his or her tiptoes (although many children without neurologic problems may also walk on their tiptoes). Children with spastic quadriplegia are more likely to have other problems, such as cognitive disability, seizures, and problems with feeding, seeing, and speaking. Following the history and physical examination, magnetic resonance imaging of the brain is usually done to look for areas of injury or congenital problems. For those children with birth defects or metabolic problems, a genetic evaluation is often considered. Further testing may be done depending on the child's case.

Given the wide array of problems caused by cerebral palsy, an interdisciplinary approach to care is most helpful. Children may need adaptive equipment (ie, walkers or wheelchairs) to help with functioning and should

Table 9-1
Cerebral Palsy

Motor Classification	Potential Causes
Spastic hemiplegia (spasticity of half of body)	Stroke
	Infection
	Genetic or developmental problems
	Infarction (tissue death) as a complication of intraventricular hemorrhage in premature infants
Spastic diplegia (spasticity of lower extremities)	Prematurity
	Lack of blood and/or oxygen supply
	Infection
	Hormonal or metabolic problems

(continued)

Table 9-1
Cerebral Palsy (continued)

Motor Classification	Potential Causes
Spastic quadriplegia (spasticity of upper and lower extremities)	Lack of blood and/or oxygen supply
	Infection
	Hormonal or metabolic problems
	Genetic or developmental problems
Athetoid/choreoathetoid/extrapyramidal (increased tone in upper and lower extremities, abnormal movements)	Asphyxia/no oxygen supply
	Kernicterus (neurologic damage from high levels of bilirubin in neonatal jaundice)
	Mitochondrial disorders
	Genetic/metabolic problems

receive physical therapy, occupational therapy, and speech therapy, if needed. In addition to the pediatrician and neurologist, physical medicine doctors or orthopedists may be involved for the management of spasticity. There are some medications that help treat spasticity, such as baclofen or even botulinum toxin injections (Botox [Allergan Inc] is for more than just a pretty face that's free of wrinkles). An initial ophthalmology assessment is warranted given the increased incidence of eye problems, such as strabismus.

ELECTRICAL BRAINSTORM

Seizures are a relatively common neurologic disorder that occurs in about 10% of children.[1] Seizures can be triggered by something going on in the body, such as a high fever, infection, toxins, head trauma, or lack of oxygen to brain, or as a result of epilepsy, a neurologic condition with disturbed brain activity that causes unprovoked seizures.

There are many different seizure types and it is important to get an accurate description of the episode to gain some insight into the cause or be able to better manage the seizure. First, figure out whether the seizure was focal (involving only part of the brain, also known as a partial seizure) or if it was generalized. Partial seizures can further be categorized into simple or complex. During a simple seizure, the child remains awake and is aware of what is going on as opposed to the more complicated complex seizure, where the child loses consciousness and cannot recall what happened. Most commonly, simple partial seizures have a motor component, which is limited to one part of the body (such as the face, neck, arms, or legs), and some can even look like tics. Simple partial seizures can also be experiencing sounds, smells, visual changes, or even hallucinations. Complex partial seizures usually have a motor component as well, but the child is unaware (of course, this distinction can be challenging depending on the age of the child). Some examples of complex partial seizures are lip smacking, chewing, picking or pulling at something, rubbing objects, or making other non-purposeful movements.

Generalized seizures also come in a variety of types, depending on the movement, and may or may not include convulsions. Tonic-clonic seizures are the most common seizures and are most frequently depicted as a convulsive seizure. Also known as grand mal seizures, these cause movements all over the body, starting with the tonic phase (muscles tense up) followed by the clonic phase (muscles contract and relax, causing convulsions). The person is not aware of what is going on and usually takes a while to return to normal because all of the brain activity leads to drowsiness or a post-seizure nap—more formally known as the postictal period. Absence seizures (not such a grand show, as they are called *petit mal seizures*) are a form of generalized seizures without convulsions causing brief periods of blanking out or staring into space. These episodes can be very brief and hard to recognize, but the child may have trouble in school because of frequent attacks during the day. Aside from tonic-clonic and absence seizures, other types of generalized seizures include tonic, clonic, myoclonic (muscle twitching or jerking), atonic (lapse in muscle tone, "drop attacks"), or a combination of these moves.

There are also seizures that are unclassified because it is not known whether they are focal or generalized. An example of this is infantile spasms, or West syndrome. These seizures typically begin between age 4 and 8 months in a developmentally delayed child as spasms of the neck, trunk, and extremities. These seizures are more difficult to manage. If you are one of the few people who understands the squiggles on electroencephalography to look at brain activity, infantile spasms has a characteristic pattern known as hypsarrhythmia—a fun word for a not-so-fun condition.

Treatment for seizures is dependent on the cause. If a seizure is caused by low blood sugar or an abnormal sodium level, correcting the imbalance will suffice. However, in cases when the underlying cause cannot be corrected or in recurrent seizures from epilepsy, many children are managed with anticonvulsant medications. A persistent seizure (lasting more than 20 to 30 minutes) or back-to-back seizures are described as status epilepticus, which is a medical emergency that requires close monitoring in an intensive care unit and medication to break the seizure (often a medication class called benzodiazepines, such as Valium [Roche Products Inc., diazepam]) no matter what caused the seizure initially.

Now that you feel like your brain has uncontrolled electrical activity learning about seizure types, we will move to a specific case of seizure: febrile seizures. Febrile seizures are the most common seizures in childhood and occur in 2% to 5% of young children, most commonly between ages 6 months and 6 years.[2] A febrile seizure is a seizure that is associated with—you guessed it—a fever. These seizures are also split into simple and complex. A simple febrile seizure is generalized, lasts less than 15 minutes, and does not happen again in 24 hours. For an otherwise healthy child who experiences a simple febrile seizure, his or her risk for future epilepsy is just slightly higher than the risk of other children (about 1%).[3] However, a child who has a simple febrile seizure is at risk for having another febrile seizure, and the risk of future epilepsy in children with multiple febrile seizures is slightly more elevated. Complex febrile seizures require a more complicated approach. These seizures are typically prolonged (>15 minutes), have some focal component (not generalized), or happen more than once in 24 hours. In the case of complex febrile seizures, additional evaluation is needed to look for a cause.

Although most children have a febrile seizure in the setting of a viral infection, it is important to inquire about the symptoms or signs of serious illnesses that can also cause seizures, such as an infection of the central nervous system. This could include meningitis (inflammation of the lining of the brain), encephalitis (inflammation of the brain), or meningoencephalitis (if the inflammation involves both the meninges and brain). It is important to recognize these life-threatening conditions promptly given the devastating complications. Inflammation of the central nervous system is typically caused by a virus or bacteria but can also occur with disorders other than infections (ie, lupus); however, we will not cover all of the causes in this little book because there are bigger books that go over that.

BAD HEAD DAY

Headaches are a common pediatric complaint, occasionally giving providers a bit of a headache. Although they are not fun to experience and occasionally interfere with functioning, it is uncommon for headaches to be caused by a dangerous problem. However, a thorough evaluation should be done to rule out the bad stuff in certain cases.

Migraine headaches occur relatively frequently in the pediatric population. Children will often have a family history of migraines, so this is an important question to ask. A migraine without an aura is the most common, usually causing throbbing pain on one side of the head in the temporal area, although the pain can be frontal. The pain interferes with activity and the child may have to lie down in a dark room. A child may also have sensitivity to light or noise, nausea, vomiting, or even abdominal pain, although these do not have to be present. Migraine with an aura is a headache preceded by visual changes, such as blurry vision, scotoma (area of abnormal vision), flickering lights, or other nonvisual symptoms.

Sometimes migraines can have particular triggers, so keeping a journal, or a "headache diary," can be helpful. Potential triggers include stress, lack of sleep, menses, certain foods, and dehydration. Treatment for migraines includes lifestyle changes (avoiding triggers, staying hydrated, having a good sleep schedule, managing stress) in addition to pain control. Acetaminophen and ibuprofen can be effective pain relievers in children, although triptans (class of medication, such as sumatriptan) are occasionally prescribed as an abortive medication in older children. Medication works best when taken at the onset of the headache. In addition, medications to help with nausea and vomiting are also prescribed. If migraines are frequent, severe, or interfere with quality of life and functioning, prophylactic medication to prevent headaches may be warranted. These medications are taken daily to prevent migraines from occurring. Some providers also recommend daily vitamin supplementation (such as magnesium or vitamin B_2), which can help prevent migraines.

Tension headaches also occur commonly, and more so in older children. The pain is typically in the frontal region and is usually described as aching as opposed to throbbing. These headaches occur during the school day or may be associated with a stressful event and often worsen throughout the day. Tension headaches do not have the associated symptoms of migraines. Headaches can also be caused by depression, so children may have associated trouble sleeping, mood changes, a change in appetite, or a loss of interest in being social or participating in usual activities. Another type of headache that can appear similar to tension headaches can be caused by drinking a lot of caffeine or stopping caffeine abruptly. In addition, if a child is taking frequent analgesics (acetaminophen, ibuprofen), it is possible to get a rebound headache (or medication overuse headache), so stopping the medication will eventually lead to headache relief.

Less frequently, headaches can be a sign of something more serious and scary, such as increased intracranial pressure, brain tumors, bleeding in the brain, or blood vessel abnormalities (such as an arteriovenous malformation), infections (meningitis, encephalitis or cerebral abscess), or chronic lead poisoning. Pseudotumor cerebri is increased intracranial pressure and the cause is often not known. It occurs mostly in adolescents and can be associated with obesity, certain medications, or even oral contraceptive pills. The pressure in the brain is measured from the cerebrospinal fluid by a lumbar puncture. In other cases, head imaging may be required to rule out an organic problem. Warning signs that the headache may be caused by something more serious include the following:

- Any abnormality on the neurological physical examination (such as weakness or lack of coordination or balance)
- Papilledema (swelling of the optic disc on fundoscopic examination, suggesting increased intracranial pressure)
- Worst headache of one's life or new-onset severe headaches
- An abrupt change in the type of headache
- Worsening headaches, in frequency or severity, over a period of days
- Headaches that wake a child up from sleep or early morning headache (can be a sign of increased intracranial pressure) or positional headache
- Weight loss
- Fever (infection, such as meningitis, encephalitis, abscess)

- Growth changes
- Seizures
- Loss of consciousness or altered mental status

In children with concerning signs or symptoms, further evaluation is warranted to rule out organic causes of headache.

When a fever is present with a headache, it may just be the flu, but central nervous system infections should be considered. Infections include meningitis (inflammation of the meninges or lining of the brain), encephalitis (inflammation of the brain), or brain abscess. Possible symptoms include, but are not limited to, headache, nausea or vomiting, fever, light sensitivity, neck pain or rigidity, back pain, or seizures. A lumbar puncture to evaluate the cerebrospinal fluid is usually required for diagnosis, or head imaging in the case of an abscess. Viruses, bacteria, fungi, or parasites can all cause infections, and infections can rarely be caused by extension from another site, such as a sinus infection. Some of the many causes of meningitis are listed in Table 9-2. There are also noninfectious causes of meningitis, such as malignancy or systemic lupus erythematosus, but we will focus on the infectious causes.

Bacterial meningitis, in particular, can do a lot of damage and is life threatening. In newborns, meningitis is more common so a fever is always taken very seriously as a potential sign of a serious infection and can be accompanied by poor feeding or lethargy. Group B *streptococci* and *Escherichia coli* are the most common causes of neonatal meningitis. Infections with Group B *streptococci* are the reason why pregnant women are tested for this bacterium and receive antibiotics prior to delivery of the baby if positive. Neonatal infection with herpes simplex virus is also important to consider because it can have devastating neurologic consequences. In children, *pneumoniae* is the most common cause of meningitis,

Table 9-2
Infectious Causes of Meningitis and
Meningoencephalitis

Viruses

- Enteroviruses (most commonly coxsackievirus, echovirus)
- Herpes virus (Epstein-Barr virus, cytomegalovirus, herpes simplex virus, human herpes virus type 6, Varicella-zoster virus)
- Arboviruses (St. Louis encephalitis virus, West Nile virus, Eastern equine encephalitis virus, Western equine encephalitis virus, California encephalitis viruses)
- Influenza
- Parvovirus B_{19}
- Adenovirus
- Lymphocytic choriomeningitis virus
- Rabies
- Parainfluenza
- Rhinovirus
- Rotaviruses
- Coronaviruses
- Measles
- Mumps
- Rubella
- HIV

Bacteria

- *Neisseria meningitidis*
- *Streptococcus pneumoniae*
- *Escherichia coli*
- *Streptococcus agalactiae* (Group B *streptococcus*)
- *Haemophilus influenzae*
- *Staphylococcus aureus*

(continued)

Table 9-2
Infectious Causes of Meningitis and Meningoencephalitis (continued)

- *Listeria monocytogenes*
- *Pasteurella multocida*
- *Mycobacterium tuberculosis* (tuberculosis)
- *Leptospira* (leptospirosis)
- *Treponema pallidum* (syphilis)
- *Borrelia burgdorferi* (Lyme disease)
- *Nocardia* species
- *Brucella* species
- *Bartonella* species (cat-scratch disease)
- *Rickettsia rickettsiae*
  (Rocky Mountain spotted fever)
- *Rickettsia prowazekii* (typhus)
- *Ehrlichia canis*
- *Coxiella burnetii*
- *Mycoplasma pneumoniae*
- *Mycoplasma hominis*
- *Chlamydia trachomatis*
- *Chlamydophilia psittaci*
- *Chlamydophilia pneumoniae*

Fungi

- *Coccidiomycosis*
- *Blastomycosis*
- *Cryptococcosis*
- *Histoplasmosis*
- *Candida* species
- *Aspergillus*

Parasites

- *Toxoplasma gondii* (toxoplasmosis)
- *Acanthamoeba* species
- *Naegleria fowleri*

(continued)

Table 9-2
Infectious Causes of Meningitis and Meningoencephalitis (continued)

- Malaria
- *Angiostrongylus cantonensis*
- *Gnathostoma spinigerum*
- *Baylisascaris procyonis*
- *Strongyloides stercoralis*
- *Trichinella spiralis*
- *Toxocara canis*
- *Taenia solium* (cysticercosis)
- *Paragonimus westermani*
- *Schistosoma* species
- *Fasciola* species

---

and in adolescents *meningitidis* is the most common cause and can occur in isolated cases or in outbreaks (such as in college dormitories). *Influenzae* type B is also an important cause of meningitis, although this has become less common with immunization (but should definitely be considered in inadequately immunized children). Meningitis requires prompt diagnosis, hospitalization, and urgent antibiotic treatment to prevent serious complications or death.

WHERE IS MY MIND?

Although kids can appear to be in an alternate universe, altered mental status can be a medical condition that requires prompt evaluation. Altered mental status is a change in a child's responsiveness, awareness, or consciousness and can include a wide range of sensorium, from confusion, disorientation, or trouble with memory to unconsciousness and coma. The Glasgow Coma Scale (Table 9-3) is an objective way to measure the state of consciousness, providing a score from 3 to 15 and coma being a score less than 8. The total score is the sum from the scores in the three categories of eye response, verbal response, and motor response.

There is a long list of causes, so the child's history is critical because there may be clues, such as certain preceding symptoms, like a fever (infection or certain medications more likely) or an open bottle of pills. Altered mental status can happen suddenly (perhaps trauma or bleeding) or be more gradual (infection, toxin, or metabolic changes). Altered mental status can come from toxins or poisoning (ie, lead, carbon monoxide poisoning, family member's medication, overdose), drugs (a big one in adolescents, including alcohol, amphetamines, ecstasy, cocaine, marijuana, mushrooms, LSD, salvia, benzodiazepines, narcotics...the list goes on), electrolyte abnormalities or metabolic changes (ie, low blood sugar, abnormal sodium levels, or changes due to liver or kidney failure), heat stroke, brain tumor, intracranial bleeding, extreme blood pressure changes, or diabetic ketoacidosis (a serious complication of type 1 diabetes).

REFERENCES

1. Kliegman R, Nelson W. *Nelson Textbook Of Pediatrics.* Philadelphia, PA: Elsevier/Saunders; 2011.
2. Febrile seizures: clinical practice guideline for the long-term management of the child with simple febrile seizures. *Pediatrics.* 2008;121(6):1281-1286.
3. Nelson KB, Ellenberg JH. Predictors of epilepsy in children who have experienced febrile seizures. *N Engl J Med.* 1976;295:1029-33.

Table 9-3
Glasgow Coma Scale

Behavior	Response	Adjustment for Children Younger than 5 Years	Score
Eye opening response	Spontaneous		4
	Open to speech		3
	Open to pain		2
	No response		1
Best verbal response	Oriented to person, place, time	Appropriate words/phrases or appropriate cooing or smiling	5
	Confused	Inappropriate words/consolable crying	4
	Inappropriate words	Persistent inappropriate crying or screaming	3
	Incomprehensible sounds	Grunts or agitated/restless	2
	No response	No response	1

(continued)

Table 9-3
Glasgow Coma Scale (continued)

Behavior	Response	Adjustment for Children Younger than 5 Years	Score
Best motor response	Obeys and follows commands		6
	Moves to localized pain		5
	Withdraws from pain		4
	Abnormal flexion (decorticate)		3
	Abnormal extension (decerebrate)		2
	No response		1
Total score	Best response		15
	Comatose		<8

Chapter 10

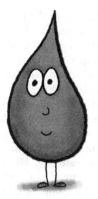

It's in My Blood (Hematology/ Oncology)

The blood is composed of numerous different things, including water, proteins, nutrients, and cells that have various jobs within the body. Hematology (the study of blood) and oncology (the study of cancers) are a single specialty within pediatrics and represent some of the most feared medical problems for children and their families.

Steiner MJ, Kimple KS. *The Little Book of Pediatrics: Infants to Teens and Everything in Between* (pp 139-144). © 2016 Taylor & Francis Group.

LOOKIN' A LITTLE PALE

Anemia is a decrease in the amount of hemoglobin present in your bloodstream. The hemoglobin and the red blood cells that carry it are responsible for carrying the majority of oxygen that your body needs to function and survive. All blood cells are generally made in the bone marrow, or middle parts, of certain bones. Healthy bone marrow and normal nutrition levels allow the body to replenish cells as they die and are used up by the body. Decreases in hemoglobin that are immediate and fast, such as might happen with severe, uncontrolled bleeding, are life threatening. Hemoglobin levels that slowly decrease over time can lead to problems with brain development in young children and shortness of breath and fatigue for everyone.

The most common type of anemia in the world is due to a deficiency of iron in the body. Hemoglobin is largely made up from iron, and low iron levels decrease the body's ability to create hemoglobin. Decreases in iron can be due to chronic, slow blood loss, as happens in certain parasite infections, or, more commonly, due to inadequate iron intake. Somewhat surprisingly, despite increasing amounts of obesity in children in the United States, the rates of iron deficiency have not decreased, probably because the highly caloric foods contributing to obesity are generally not very rich in nutrients. In addition, for infants breastmilk is not very rich in iron. Preventing iron deficiency early in life is the reason that rice cereal sold for babies is heavily enriched with iron. Up to 20% of poor children in the United States between ages 1 and 2 years have iron deficiency, and this lack of iron has been demonstrated to cause permanent changes in adult intelligence and cognitive ability, even if the deficiency is not severe enough to cause a decrease in the hemoglobin concentration.[1]

There are many other causes of anemia in children, such as genetic changes in the red blood cell structure (eg, sickle cell anemia). In addition, children with chronic diseases can frequently develop anemia, as happens with bowel problems like IBD where blood leaking into the stool causes a decrease in and lack of iron and inflammation keeps the bone marrow from keeping up with making new blood. In diseases of kidney function, a key hormone that stimulates the bone marrow to make hemoglobin decreases and anemia can develop. Finally, in the most feared cases, a cancer that affects the bone marrow, such as leukemia, replaces all of the natural cells and stops the body from making enough new cells. Because of the problems associated with iron deficiency anemia and the potential serious diseases, anemia should always be taken seriously in children.

RUNS LIKE A RIVER: BLEEDING AND PLATELET DISORDERS

Regulating bleeding is a complex series of events that includes cells called *platelets* and various proteins in the body. Although the cells are made in the bone marrow, the proteins are made in a variety of places, including the blood vessels themselves and the liver. The spleen is an organ in the abdomen that helps clean up dead or used blood cells and filters other things out of the blood. Low platelets can develop for a variety of reasons but all of them are potentially serious. A somewhat common cause of low platelets in otherwise well children is something called *idiopathic thrombocytopenic purpura*. This scientific name explains that we do not know why it develops, but it causes low platelet counts and spontaneous small spots of bleeding into the skin (purpura or petechiae). This happens because children make antibodies or proteins that bind to the platelets, causing the platelets to get caught and collected by the spleen. Other causes of low platelets are also associated with more severe systemic diseases, such as other autoimmune disorders or severe infections. Like with anemia, low platelets can also be an early sign of blood cancers like leukemia.

The most common genetically inherited bleeding disorder is von Willebrand's disease. This is a problem with one of the proteins that starts the cascade that leads to blood clotting. Bleeding with this disorder is usually mild but may manifest in heavy, regular menstrual bleeding or frequent nose bleeds, although both of these things are more commonly due to other reasons. There are also severe bleeding disorders that can be inherited, such as hemophilia. This disease also lacks a protein in the clotting cascade; however, if this protein is totally absent, then the bleeding is severe, with spontaneous bleeding into the joints and other spaces in the body. When children are missing all of this protein, they need to take expensive medications that replace the protein to avoid severe complications of this disease.

THE BIG 'C': CHILDHOOD CANCERS

Childhood cancers are probably the most feared childhood disease. However, for many of these cancers, this is slowly becoming inaccurate as treatments get better and better. For example, some types of leukemia in children now have 95% survival rates.[2] Despite all of the advances, there is also great hope that we are still early in our understanding of cancer, and it is likely that in 20 years the treatments will be totally different than the regimens of today. Table 10-1 provides the most common types of cancer in childhood by age of the child.

Table 10-1
Most Common Childhood Cancers by Age,
Likelihood of Survival With New Treatments

Cancer Type	Age Range	Likelihood of Survival in 5 Years
Leukemia	All ages	Best types of leukemia: 90% or higher. Rate is variable.
Brain tumors	All ages	Highly variable survival
Lymphoma	More common in older children and adolescents	80% to 95%
Neuroblastoma	More common in younger children	Vary from 50% to 95%
Sarcoma of soft tissues	Relatively stable in all ages	Variable based on tumor type, size, and location
Wilms tumor (kidney)	From age 1 to 10 years	85% to 90%
Bone tumors	Most common in older children/ adolescents	If local: 70% to 85%; if metastasized: 20% to 30%

HOW IS CANCER TREATED?

Cancer is generally treated in one of four ways, and these are usually combined in treatment regimens.

First, many cancers can be "cut out" surgically. This is particularly true for cancers of an organ, such as the skin, kidneys, brain, or adrenal glands. This does not work for blood cancers like leukemia or lymphoma, where the cancer circulates throughout the body. Second, cancer is often directly destroyed by using radiation, which can poison cancer cells and cause them to die. New machines and techniques can focus the radiation in very small, specific areas. Chemotherapy is the third, and most common type of cancer treatment and, in general, can be thought of as a medication that is taken up and kills rapidly or abnormally producing cells. The fourth, relatively newer type of cancer treatment is called a *bone marrow transplant*. In this type of therapy, medications are used to kill off all of the abnormal cells (and often most of the good bone marrow cells) and then new cells are given to the person either from his or her own body before the medication or from another person. Sometimes umbilical cord cells from newborn babies can be donated to create new bone marrow. All of these treatments have risks and side effects, including making people more likely to get infections, skin and mouth sores, baldness, and other types of cancer.

REFERENCES

1. Brotanek J, Gosz J, Weitzman M, Flores G. Secular trends in the prevalence of iron deficiency among US toddlers, 1976-2002. *Arch Pediatr Adolesc Med*. 2008;162(4):374.
2. Matloub Y, Bostrom B, Hunger S et al. Escalating intravenous methotrexate improves event-free survival in children with standard-risk acute lymphoblastic leukemia: a report from the children's oncology group. *Blood*. 2011;118(2):243-251.

Chapter 11

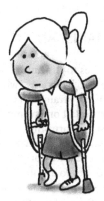

Not so Humerus (Musculoskeletal)

Let's face it—little kids can be rough on their bodies. Although their bones can withstand a bump or two, orthopedic injuries are a relatively common consequence. In addition, more student athletes may be following the "no pain, no gain" training plan, leading to overuse injuries or even ignoring injuries that will result in them never completely regaining normal function. Problems with the bones and joints may not always result from trauma, and kids may have a bone to pick with other

Steiner MJ, Kimple KS. *The Little Book of Pediatrics: Infants to Teens and Everything in Between* (pp 145-153).
© 2016 Taylor & Francis Group.

causes, like infection, cancer, or disorders of the immune systems affecting the joints.

SPRAINS, STRAINS, AND BONE MOBILITY

Most acute injuries to the musculoskeletal system are sprains (injury to the ligaments, which connect bones to bones or to joints), strains (injury to the muscle or tendon, which connects bone to muscle), or contusions (injury to soft tissue or bruising). Fractures of the bone can also occur, especially in growing children, and diagnosis and treatment require consideration of the differences in growing bones to ensure that kids can continue to play and keep growing without issues.

Depending on the location, sprains can result in pain, swelling, limping, bruising, or even instability, depending on the severity of the injury. Sprains get a grade depending on how bad they are, and patients may eventually graduate to the care of an orthopedist. A grade 1 sprain is a more mild injury with some ligament fibers torn but otherwise a good, strong joint. A grade 2 sprain has a little bit of give to the joint because more ligament fibers are torn. A grade 3 sprain means that the ligament is completely torn and the joint is loose as a result. Strains are also on the grading system, depending on how much damage is done to the tendon or muscle. Grade 1 strains result in mild to moderate pain and not much weakness. Grade 2 strains have more pain and some weakness in muscle strength. Grade 3 strains, like sprains, describe a completely torn muscle or tendon that results in significant weakness. For most sprains and strains, a little RICE (Rest, Ice, Compression, and Elevation) may be all that is needed, along with a little pain relief from an anti-inflammatory medication, such as ibuprofen or naproxen. More severe injuries (ie, tears of the anterior cruciate ligament of the knee) require medical care and potentially surgery. In any case, exercises to improve strength, flexibility, and function are important and some kids may even benefit from physical therapy.

Given the immature, growing bones of a child, damage to the bone is more likely than injury of the ligaments or joints in younger children. However, fractures in children heal more quickly than those in adults. Fractures of the physis, or growth plate, are important to recognize because they can lead to problems with the growth plate. Fractures that involve the growth plate are classified into five groups called the Salter-Harris fracture types, described by Salter and Harris.[1] Some like to use the mnemonic, SALTER, to keep these straight:

I. S, for Slipped or Straight across

II. A, for Above

III. L, for Lower

IV. TE, for Through Everything

V. R, for Rammed

These fracture types, which can help guide treatment and prognosis, are summarized in Table 11-1.

Fractures are usually diagnosed with x-rays, although some may be tricky to see and require a trained eye. In addition, an x-ray may not show a Salter-Harris I fracture unless there is significant displacement, and the injury should be treated as a fracture if there is suspicion of a Salter-Harris I fracture that is not obvious on x-ray. Treatment of fractures involves splinting or casting, although occasionally fractures may need to be reduced (a nicer word for pulling bones back into place, usually with sedation and pain medication) or even fixed together in the operating room.

Broken bones can lead to complications, such as damage to the tissue, nerves, or vessels around the injury. In addition to treating the fracture, providers should make sure there is good blood flow, sensation, and motor

Table 11-1
Salter-Harris Classification

Salter-Harris Type	What It Is	Picture
I	Separation through physis or growth plate	
II	Fracture through portion of physis, extends through metaphysis (wider portion of long bone)	
III	Fracture through portion of physis, extending through epiphysis (end of long bone) and into joint	
IV	Fracture across the metaphysis, physis, and epiphysis (strike through the whole growth plate)	
V	Crush injury to the physis/growth plate	

Reprinted with permission from Dr. Frank Gaillard, via Wikimedia Commons.

function (yes, there is pain, but things are still in working order). One serious complication that requires prompt medical attention is compartment syndrome, usually of the arm or leg. The extremities are divided into compartments, hence the name. If there is not enough room for the swelling or bleeding from the injury within the walls of thick fibrous tissue, pressure builds up and leads to the potential five Ps: pain (usually out of proportion to injury), paresthesias (tingling or abnormal sensation), pallor (loss of color), paralysis (I can't move my toes!), and pulselessness (no pulse, blood flow is compromised). Most of these signs do not occur because they are very late findings. Usually, pain is the only symptom early on, so it can be hard to diagnose. The pressure can be measured with a device by inserting a needle into the compartment, although some orthopedic surgeons may just go ahead and treat. Treatment for compartment syndrome is an emergent trip to the operating room to relieve the pressure by cutting the fibrous tissue, otherwise known as a fasciotomy. Another type of urgent fracture that requires immediate evaluation is a supracondular fracture, or fracture of the distal humerus right above the elbow.

It is also important to consider non-accidental trauma, or child abuse, in children with traumatic injuries. Fractures that are particularly suspicious are femur fractures in children not yet walking, fractures or spiral fractures of the long bones (require a lot of force), posterior rib fractures, and corner fractures (small corner of the bone broken off). No one type of fracture means definitive child abuse, but the patient's history is critical to figuring out what happened and whether the injury is consistent with the explained mechanism and whether the child needs further evaluation.

HIP HOP

There are many causes of limb and joint pain that are not preceded by injury, such as infections or rheumatologic disorders. Joint pain may be accompanied by swelling or fluid within the joint and could have redness with infection or significant inflammation. We will not cover all of the causes of joint pain, some of which are benign and others that can be very serious and require prompt attention. Table 11-2 summarizes many of the causes of joint pain, in no particular order.

Bacterial infection of the joint, known as septic arthritis, can cause severe joint pain that usually affects one joint, such as the hip, knee, or ankle. Children typically develop symptoms acutely with a fever and a red, hot, swollen, and painful joint and are resistant to any movement of the joint. The infection typically travels to the joint through blood vessels or the adjacent bone, but sometimes a child may have a preceding injury to the skin, allowing bacteria to enter. The most common bacteria that cause septic arthritis are *Staphylococcus aureus* in children and adolescents, although *Neisseria gonorrhoeae* can occur in this latter group. *Kingella kingae* is also an important cause, typically seen in children in daycare younger than age 5 years. These children need prompt medical evaluation to prevent complications and damage to the joint, including examination of the joint fluid and intravenous antibiotics to treat the infection.

When a bacterial infection occurs in the bone, it is called *osteomyelitis*, and this may accompany septic arthritis or occur on its own. Like septic arthritis, the infection spreads to the bone through the bloodstream or directly from trauma, such as a puncture wound or fracture. Symptoms can be vague but a fever may be present and older children will refuse to bear weight. Laboratory studies are typically consistent with inflammation and a

Table 11-2
Causes of Joint Pain in Children

- Avascular necrosis/Legg-Calvé-Perthes disease
- Slipped capital femoral epiphysis
- Toxic synovitis
- Acute rheumatic fever
- Reiter syndrome (reactive arthritis)
- Trauma or overuse syndrome
- Leukemia
- Neuroblastoma
- Bleeding disorders (hemophilia, sickle cell disease)
- Rickets
- Serum sickness
- Septic arthritis (with or without osteomyelitis)
- Lyme arthritis
- Viral-associated arthritis (eg, parvovirus)
- Tumor (eg, osteosarcoma)
- Idiopathic pain syndromes
- Systemic rheumatologic disorders (juvenile idiopathic arthritis, systemic lupus erythematosus)
- Kawasaki disease
- Henoch–Schönlein purpura

blood culture might show the organism responsible for the infection, but not always. X-rays will show eventual changes, but if early in the infection process, magnetic resonance imaging (MRI) is better for diagnosing osteomyelitis. Like septic arthritis, S aureus is the most common organism, although again there are a variety of bacteria that can be the cause, and children are treated with intravenous antibiotics initially and then oral antibiotics to complete a long course.

Transient synovitis is a relatively common cause of hip pain or limp that is benign but important to distinguish from more serious causes of pain, such as septic arthritis. Transient synovitis typically affects children between ages 3 and 8 years and may follow a recent upper respiratory infection. The child who presents with acute hip pain or a limp will usually have mildly decreased range of motion in the hip, especially when rotating the hip inward. Keep in mind that hip pain in children can also present as pain in the knee, groin, or thigh. X-rays are typically normal, but an ultrasound of the hip may reveal fluid in the hip joint, called an *effusion*. To distinguish transient synovitis from other more serious causes like septic arthritis (bacterial infection of the joint), many times the fluid from the hip is removed with a needle and sent to the lab to determine whether it is an effusion typical of this illness or whether the fluid is more like pus, which suggests septic arthritis.

Another cause of hip or knee pain in children to keep in mind is slipped capital femoral epiphysis. The exact cause is not known, but it is classically seen in adolescent boys, and obesity is a big risk factor. The head of the femur (capital) slips from the growth plate (epiphysis), leading to pain (hip or referred knee pain) and/or a limp. To apply the exciting knowledge gained previously, slipped capital femoral epiphysis is a Salter-Harris type I fracture. The affected leg may also appear turned out and there is difficulty turning the leg inward at the hip. Diagnosis is made using pelvic x-rays, and the head of the femur is described as ice cream melting off the cone. Orthopedic surgeons get involved to pin the ice cream back on the cone in the operating room. Untreated, the bone can die from lack of blood flow or it can lead to osteoarthritis, pain, or trouble walking.

Because so much is happening with the hip, let's talk about idiopathic avascular necrosis of the hip, otherwise known as Legg-Calvé-Perthes disease. For some unknown reason (which is why it is called *idiopathic*), the femoral head does not get enough blood supply, causing hip damage from bone death and can interfere with growth. Children are typically between ages 4 and 8 years and present with a limp, perhaps mild pain in the thigh or knee (where pain is referred), and decreased hip motion. Although it can be diagnosed with x-rays, it may not be seen initially, so if there is high suspicion, MRI or a bone scan may reveal avascular necrosis. How well the child does varies on when it occurs, and some children do well without treatment, others require symptomatic treatment, and others may need surgery.

Developmental dysplasia of the hip (DDH), formally known as congenital dislocation of the hip, is a disorder that is worth bringing up briefly. Risk factors include a female infant, family history of DDH, first-born child, or breech position in utero. Providers examine the hips carefully during infancy for any clicks or clunks that would suggest a problem. For the most part, DDH is diagnosed clinically or with a hip ultrasound, although x-ray can be used in older infants. If a child is at risk for DDH, a screening ultrasound at approximately age 6 to 8 weeks can also be done. Treatment is usually a Pavlik harness—a bulky contraption that holds the hips in the correct position to encourage normal growth and development of the hip.

REFERENCE

1. Salter RB, Harris WR. Injuries involving the epiphyseal plate. *J Bone Joint Surg Am.* 1963;45(3):587–622.

Chapter 12

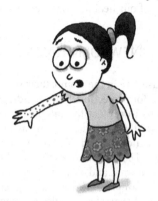

Itchy, Itchy, Scratchy, Scratchy: What's That Rashy Rashy (Dermatology)

The skin is the largest organ in the body and is critically important for body functions, including fluid

Steiner MJ, Kimple KS. *The Little Book of Pediatrics: Infants to Teens and Everything in Between* (pp 155-164).
© 2016 Taylor & Francis Group.

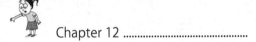

maintenance and immunity. It is also the "window to the world" for others to view our body and becomes uniquely part of our health, looks, and identity.

NEWBORN RASHES

When fetuses are in the womb, their skin is covered in amniotic fluid for protection, but immediately after birth the skin begins to protect the infant. Infants, especially those born after their due date, often having peeling skin at birth. This is normal and does not need to be treated. There are several common rashes that newborns develop, and most are normal and resolve with time as the skin matures. One example of this has a very scary sounding name but is totally harmless. Erythema toxicum are small collections of eosinophils in the middle of a red bump and often appear for 1 to 2 days after birth in full-term babies. Sebaceous gland hyperplasia is blockages of normal skin pores with sebum, or a waxy whitish substance. This is particularly common, and almost universal in a very fine way, around the nose of newborns. Milia are small 1- to 2-mm firm wax balls that are trapped under the most superficial layer of skin. Occasionally, these can be spotted on newborn skin. Miliaria rubra are small reddish bumps that occur when blocked pores get irritated and inflamed. Some people call this "prickly heat," and it can occur throughout childhood but is particularly common on the immature skin of infants. This is often confused with newborn acne, which includes small pustules. This kind of acne in the days and weeks after birth does not scar like teenager acne can. Lastly, seborrhea starts for some infants in the first few weeks of life and usually consists of scaling (sometimes thick and hard) on the scalp and fine scales around the eyes. Seborrhea can also include redness and bumps on the cheeks, around the ears, and deep in the skin creases on the arms and legs.

All of these skin conditions generally resolve on their own without any treatment and do not cause long-term problems. However, in severe or unique cases, there are treatments that can be tried.

ECZEMA OR ATOPIC DERMATITIS

This dry inflammatory skin condition is one of the most common chronic skin conditions of childhood. In essence, the problem with this condition is a chronic lack of skin hydration accompanied by itchiness and inflammation. Over time, the skin becomes thickened, scarred, and discolored. The skin then flares up and worsens when there are other inflammatory conditions, such as skin infections or allergies. For some children, this is a mild illness and is mostly present in younger children in the winter when the air is drier. For other children, this is a severe chronic condition that requires strong immunosuppressant medication taken orally and skin care multiple times per day to control. Most children fall somewhere in between these two cases and can control the disease with some minimal daily attention and other medications during exacerbations.

Fun Facts: Eczema often gets worse in the winter and this might be due to dry air. Why is the air in our homes drier in the winter? More water can be suspended in warm expanded air, and the humidity report from the weatherman often only reports the relative humidity—not the absolute humidity. So when they say 70% relative humidity in the winter that is still less water in the air than 70% relative humidity on a hot summer day. Therefore, a box of air in the winter would tend to have less water in it than the same size box of air in the summer. As that relatively dry air then comes into our house and is heated, it expands further with no additional water added to it. This makes for super dry conditions in many houses in the winter.

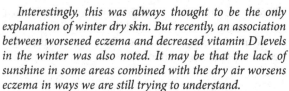

Interestingly, this was always thought to be the only explanation of winter dry skin. But recently, an association between worsened eczema and decreased vitamin D levels in the winter was also noted. It may be that the lack of sunshine in some areas combined with the dry air worsens eczema in ways we are still trying to understand.

Treatment of eczema in children combines daily care with special care during exacerbations or worsening. Children with moderate and persistent eczema should bathe with warm, but not hot, water every other day. No soap or minimal gentle soap should be used to avoid excessive drying of the skin. After bathing, they should dab the skin with a towel instead of rubbing the skin, which can activate the inflammation signals in the skin. Immediately after bathing and at least twice per day when not bathing, parents should help children apply emollients or oil-based ointments that trap moisture inside the skin to all affected areas. Petroleum jelly is a particularly good and cheap emollient. Keeping skin moisturized, soft, and smooth helps calm the inflammation and the disease. Regardless of how mild the eczema is, most children will have periods with some flare-ups where the skin gets rough, thickened, and itchy. Scratching the skin during this time makes the skin even more irritated and creates a vicious itch-scratch cycle that continues to worsen. In this setting, it is important to use a medication to decrease the itchiness and calm the inflammation. The best medications to do this are topical steroid ointments. The mildest of these can be bought over the counter, such as 1% hydrocortisone, but the more powerful medications require a prescription. Caution needs to be used with the more powerful medications, and the prescribing doctor should tell you where you can use it and for how long.

RINGWORM

Ringworm is a relatively simple and harmless skin infection caused by an infestation with a small fungus. This infection can occur anywhere on the body, including the scalp, body, arms, legs, genital area, and feet. The classic lesion is a round area with a raised border filled with small red bumps. When it is in the scalp, the hairs in that area often fall out or are broken off, causing local partial baldness. In the groin, it can spread quickly due to the damp warmth and cover the genitals and groin area. On the feet, it usually consists of peeling and flaking between the toes, otherwise known as athlete's foot. Ringworm is relatively simple to treat and can usually be cured by applying an anti-fungal cream twice per day until the rash is gone. Most of these creams are available over-the-counter as "Athlete's Foot Cream," but they will generally work for any body part. However, when ringworm is in the scalp, it is slightly more difficult to treat because of all the hair follicles, so people then need to take an oral medication for 2 to 3 months to get rid of the infection.

YEAST INFECTIONS

These infections are another common childhood infection, particularly when children are in diapers. Yeast, and *Candida* species particularly, like to grow in wet, warm places, such as in the diaper region, between rolls of skin, under the neck of a drooling baby, or in the vaginal mucosa after puberty.

This red rash is not very itchy and is relatively easy to identify because it often spares areas right next to the skin fold that are not moist, and you can often see small little red irritated bumps next to the infected site where the yeast are trying to spread. Over-the-counter topical anti-fungal medications will generally cure these infections, but prescription medications are also available.

VIRAL EXANTHEMS

Viral infections are one of the most common causes of temporary rashes. Almost all common viral infections that children get can have manifestations in the skin. Historically, measles and chickenpox were commonly discussed viral infections with important skin symptoms; however, these have become uncommon in the United States since vaccination. Currently, viruses that commonly cause skin findings are coxsackievirus, parvovirus, and human herpes virus 6. Coxsackievirus causes Hand, Foot, and Mouth disease and can cause other rash types. Parvovirus causes erythema infectiosum, or fifth disease, which classically includes a rash with strikingly red cheeks that almost look like they were recently slapped. Human herpes virus 6 (not to be confused with the herpes virus that causes herpes sexually) causes exanthema subitum or roseola. This illness usually gives young children a high fever for 3 days and then a rash begins over the trunk and rest of the body after the fever has subsided.

Parvovirus infection and roseola deserve special discussion because they are part of the febrile exanthems of childhood, and this is how parvovirus infection and rash got its name as fifth disease. The febrile exanthems that were numbered were the following:

- First disease: Measles
- Second disease: Scarlet fever
- Third disease: Rubella
- Fourth disease: Duke's disease (no longer used)

- Fifth disease: Erythema infectiosum
- Sixth disease: Roseola

This naming convention is now mostly only of historical interest, except that erythema infectiosum is still called fifth disease. Interestingly, varicella infection, or chickenpox, did not make the list of numbered febrile exanthems.

BACTERIAL SKIN INFECTIONS

Bacterial skin infections have become common in the past 15 to 20 years, in part due to the emergence of a new strain of bacteria called *Staphylococcus aureus* that has a particular predilection for skin infections.

The simplest type of bacterial skin infection is called *cellulitis*. This causes redness, warmth, and tenderness on the skin due to the bacteria and the associated immune reaction. It is generally thought that the bacteria somehow get introduced under the skin by scratching or a break in the skin and then starts to spread. This infection has a tendency to run toward the middle of the body and can creep forward over hours. The most common bacterium causing this is *Streptococcus pyogenes,* which is the same bacterium that causes strep throat. *S aureus* can also cause this type of skin infection. Antibiotics can generally stop this type of infection quickly. There is one particularly dangerous type of cellulitis called *necrotizing fasciitis* or the "flesh eating" disease. This can be caused by numerous different bacteria. This infection spreads quickly under the skin, producing severe redness, pain, and swelling. The pain with this type of infection is often worse than the body part looks, and this may be due in part to the gas that is produced by the infection and then trapped under the skin. that is often produced by this organism. This infection generally cannot be stopped solely with antibiotics and the treatment includes surgery to expose the skin on that part of the body to the air by making a series of incisions while the patient is under anesthesia.

Another type of bacterial skin infection is an abscess. Similarly to cellulitis, bacteria gets introduced under the skin but instead of running along the skin, the specific enzymes in that bacteria cause it to stay locally, degrading local tissues and causing infection-fighting white blood cells to come to that area. This creates a pocket of pus that often is tender due to the pressure as it builds up under the skin. This is the most common type of infection caused by methicillin-resistant *Staphylococcus aureus*, which has spread widely in the past two decades. The public has become very aware of this type of infection and this bacteria, but despite the widespread media attention, it is usually just a nuisance that is not life threatening. The best treatment for this type of localized bacterial skin infection is to open up the skin overlying the pocket of pus either with a needle or a small knife so that the fluid and bacteria can drain. Although doctors often treat even small infections like this with antibiotics, opening up the abscess is enough to treat it in most cases for otherwise healthy children.

ACNE

This is likely the most common of all skin rashes and is almost universally prevalent in adolescent boys and girls. The cause of acne is complex and involves the blockage of pores with sebum, or the natural oil on your skin, and is moderated in part by hormonal changes and alterations. This is then followed by a bacterial infection from a specific bacterium, called *Propionibacterium acnes*, which causes an exaggerated inflammatory reaction as the body reacts to the infection. All of these things come

Table 12-1
Has This Been Proven to Cause Acne?

Item	Has this been proven to cause acne?
Blocking pores (certain creams or anything physically blocking)	Yes
Hormones	Yes, some hormones cause changes that can increase acne
Medications	Yes, some medications can increase acne
Dirty skin	No
Cosmetics	Only if they block pores
Dairy products	Possible
Carbohydrate-rich foods	Yes
Chocolate	No
Greasy foods	No

together to cause the well-known blackheads, which are open occluded pores filled with sebum and then dust or dirt, and white heads, which are closed occluded pores that have started to recruit infection-fighting cells. In the worst cases, the infection and red inflammation can cause scarring of the skin.

Fun Facts: So many things get blamed for causing acne! Because it is a near universal condition that gets better and worse and better over time, it can be thought to be associated with a lot of different things. Table 12-1 provides a list of things that have and have not been demonstrated to actually be associated with developing acne.

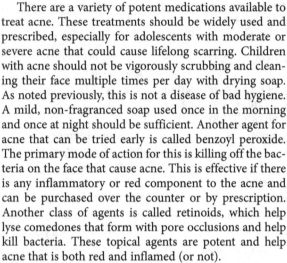

There are a variety of potent medications available to treat acne. These treatments should be widely used and prescribed, especially for adolescents with moderate or severe acne that could cause lifelong scarring. Children with acne should not be vigorously scrubbing and cleaning their face multiple times per day with drying soap. As noted previously, this is not a disease of bad hygiene. A mild, non-fragranced soap used once in the morning and once at night should be sufficient. Another agent for acne that can be tried early is called benzoyl peroxide. The primary mode of action for this is killing off the bacteria on the face that cause acne. This is effective if there is any inflammatory or red component to the acne and can be purchased over the counter or by prescription. Another class of agents is called retinoids, which help lyse comedones that form with pore occlusions and help kill bacteria. These topical agents are potent and help acne that is both red and inflamed (or not).

If acne is severe or widespread beyond the face, then many physicians will prescribe a 2- to 3-month course of an oral antibiotic from a class that also has some anti-inflammatory properties. This can help get things under control and allow the other medications to work and then eventually control acne. For adolescent girls with acne that is particularly severe or difficult to treat, oral contraceptive pills that contain estrogen and progesterone will often help to improve the acne. This is particularly true for girls who have problems such as polycystic ovarian syndrome but is also true for almost all adolescents. Finally, if there is severe acne with scarring, then a dermatologist should be involved and an oral retinoid medication can be tried. Oral retinoids must include very close monitoring of mood and some blood tests and contraception should be used because it is a teratogen.

Chapter 13

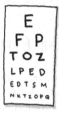

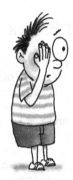

Peek-a-Boo,
I See You
(Ophthalmology)

Children often go about their days with their eyes wide open, soaking in the world around them. It is important to keep an eye out for problems during visual development because the eyes are constantly taking in external stimuli for learning. Preventing visual problems and detecting abnormalities early are critical to normal vision development. Although there is a large amount

Steiner MJ, Kimple KS. *The Little Book of Pediatrics: Infants to Teens and Everything in Between* (pp 165-174).

to learn about the little eye that will not be covered, this chapter will provide an eyeful of knowledge about vision screening and common eye complaints in children.

THE EARLIER, THE BETTER

Providers start examining the eyes in newborn infants. The eye examination differs based on the age of the child, taking into account the development of an infant and his or her ability to track or how well a toddler can cooperate or sit still. Vision screening and eye examinations occur at all ages, newborn through adolescents, during those health maintenance visits discussed in Chapter 1. Screening for vision problems in developing children is especially important given the possibility of permanent visual problems if not corrected while the eyes and brain are learning to see together, which occurs before age 8 years.

LET'S TAKE A LOOK

The eye examination is fairly similar in infants and children up to age 2 years. The examination begins by looking for any abnormality around the eye or on the eyelid. A provider can then take a peek at the eye looking for abnormalities, such as inflammation of the conjunctivae or discoloration of the normally white sclera. When using a light, the pupils should be equal on both sides and react to the light by symmetrically constricting. In addition, the cornea should reflect the light symmetrically in both eyes in relation to the pupil, called the *corneal light reflex*. Using an ophthalmoscope, the eye is then examined for any problems in the back of the eye, normally called the *red reflex*, which is the reflection of light back from the retina that makes the pupils red appearing and symmetric on both sides rather than absent, blunted, or white. This is the same appearance as the red eye sometimes seen in photographs. Seeing symmetric red eyes in the pupil on photographs is actually a good sign!

The ophthalmoscope can also be used for a fundoscopic examination to get a look at the retina, retinal blood vessels, and the optic disk, although this is not always done routinely but is important in certain cases, such as suspicion of increased intracranial pressure. In addition, the movement of the eyes is tested by seeing how an infant or child tracks an object or someone's face in all directions. A child should be able to follow with both eyes together. A child should also follow the object when one eye is covered; however, if vision in one eye differs, the infant may not like the good eye being covered and may try to move his or her head to accommodate.

Starting around age 3 years, a child should be better able to cooperate and follow instructions for visual acuity testing in addition to the previously described examination. Vision testing at this stage looks for problems seeing from refractive errors (light is not properly refracted onto retina), such as myopia (nearsightedness, far objects are blurry), hyperopia (farsightedness, near objects are blurry), or astigmatism (blurred vision from abnormal curvature of the cornea). This should be done yearly at the well-child visit using pictures on a chart in younger children and then moving to the familiar letters on a chart (called a Snellen chart; Figure 13-1) in older children. There are other tests that can be used in children, such as the HOTV test (matching the letters H, O, T, and V and the child does not have to be familiar with the alphabet) or tumbling E test (identifying the direction of the letter "E"). Children stand 20 feet from the chart and are asked to read the letters or recognize pictures (apple, house, circle, square) on the smallest readable line. Visual acuity testing is done with both eyes and then the right

Figure 13-1 Snellen chart.

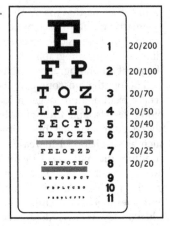

E	1	20/200
F P	2	20/100
T O Z	3	20/70
L P E D	4	20/50
P E C F D	5	20/40
E D F C Z P	6	20/30
F E L O P Z D	7	20/25
D E F P O T E C	8	20/20
L E F O D P C T	9	
F D P L T C E O	10	
P E Z O L C F T D	11	

and left eyes individually while the untested eye is covered. A normal result for visual acuity in adults is 20/20. The number 20 comes from the distance from the chart, which traditionally is 20 feet. The top number is how far away you could stand to complete the test (where you would stand to see it) and then bottom number is where someone else could stand to see the same thing. So, 20/40 means what you can see at 20 feet, other people can see from 40 feet. A child older than 3 or 4 years with any result worse than 20/40 is referred to an ophthalmologist for further evaluation. In addition, a discrepancy of two or more lines on the chart between right and left eyes is also referred for evaluation because this can lead to amblyopia (lazy eye), which is decreased vision in one eye from the brain ignoring the signal from the bad eye and thus not learning to see properly. Problems of refraction or visual acuity can be corrected with glasses— or aptly named, corrective lenses. If amblyopia is present, then patching of the good eye can be used (which is fun for driving kids crazy).

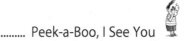

Fun Fact: Newborns can only focus about 8 to 12 inches away and vision is very blurry at first. However, they have a preference for their mother's face. The newborn's vision is estimated to be 20/800 but quickly improves to 20/50 by age 1 year.

DEVIANT BEHAVIOR

In addition to visual acuity, children are also tested for eye alignment. Strabismus (crossed eyes) is a disorder of eye alignment when the eyes do not line up or move together. An infant's eyes may intermittently wander in the first month of life while he or she is getting the hang of coordinating eye movements, but constant eye deviation should be evaluated. A child may be born with strabismus, develop one in the first 6 months of life (as in the case of congenital esotropia), or pick it up along the way. In rare cases, serious disorders can cause strabismus, such as retinoblastoma.

For the brain to get correct images, both of the eyes and the eye muscles holding them in place need to all work together. If one eye does not move with the other, then the brain gets an abnormal signal, potentially affecting vision and depth perception (since information from both eyes are coordinated to determine depth). Like refractive errors, strabismus can also lead to amblyopia from the brain ignoring the eye that is not straight, thus affecting vision in that eye and making it lazy. Therefore, recognizing and correcting strabismus early can prevent permanent vision problems, in addition to preventing problems in social interaction and self-esteem.

Strabismus is any misalignment of the eyes, but the direction of the deviated eye is also noted. Inward deviation of the eye is called *esotropia* and outward deviation is called *exotropia*. Vertical deviation can also occur, called *hypertropia* when one eye is higher or *hypotropia* when one eye is lower than the other. Occasionally, a child may even adjust his or her head position to help with the misalignment. Strabismus can occasionally be noted just by looking at the eyes but can also be detected by using the corneal light reflex (discussed previously), cover test, cover/uncover test, and the random-dot-E stereo test. The cover test is when a child fixes on a distant object and then the examiner covers one eye while looking for movement in the uncovered eye. Any dance moves in the uncovered eye are not wanted and should dance their way to the ophthalmologist for further evaluation. In addition, when the cover is taken away from the covered eye, that eye should have remained aligned. The random-dot-E test is a "game" that involves cards and polarized glasses. This test can look at how well a child can detect depth, which can be affected by strabismus or decreased vision in one eye (amblyopia). Strabismus should be referred to an ophthalmologist, where treatment consists of eyeglasses, vision therapy, and occasionally corrective surgery.

ROMPIN' WITH ROP

Premature infants are a subset of patients that require screening and serial evaluations by an ophthalmologist given the risk of retinopathy of prematurity (ROP). ROP is a disease of the eye related to the developing blood vessels of the retina. Many infants will have no visual deficits, but in severe cases, ROP can lead to visual impairment or blindness from retinal detachment.

RED-TINTED WINDOWS

There are many etiologies for a red eye, but in children, the most common is conjunctivitis, also known as "pink eye." Conjunctivitis typically comes in three types: viral, bacterial, and allergic. Viral conjunctivitis is the most common, causing redness, watery or mucoid discharge (which may be worse in the morning and improve throughout the day), or eye mattering or sticking together. It also may start in one eye and then move to the other eye within 1 to 2 days. Viral conjunctivitis is contagious and is often spread among children in daycare or school. Adenovirus or enterovirus is typically the culprit. The infection should resolve on its own and no specific treatment is required.

Viral conjunctivitis is very difficult to differentiate from bacterial conjunctivitis because both have similar symptoms. Bacterial conjunctivitis also causes eye redness and eye mattering, but the drainage is typically more purulent, or pus-like, and there may be more discomfort in the eye. However, even with all these signs, viral and bacterial conjunctivitis can be indistinguishable. A bacterial infection can also occur in an adolescent wearing contact lenses or following trauma to the eye. Common causes include *Haemophilus influenzae* and *Streptococcus pneumoniae. Neisseria gonorrhoeae* or *Chlamydia trachomatis* can cause conjunctivitis in newborns or adolescents. Ophthalmia neonatorum is a special case of bacterial conjunctivitis occurring in newborns within the first month of life, which can have serious, blinding consequences. This is caused by transmission of bacteria from the mother, such as chlamydia, gonorrhea, or *Staphylococcus aureus*, and requires antibiotic treatment. Ophthalmia neonatorum is not seen as often now with maternal screening for sexually transmitted infections and erythromycin or silver nitrate prophylaxis at birth.

> **Table 13-1**
> Causes of a Red Eye in Children
>
> - Viral conjunctivitis
> - Bacterial conjunctivitis
> - Ophthalmia neonatorum/neonatal conjunctivitis
> - Allergic conjunctivitis
> - Keratitis
> - Endophthalmitis
> - Anterior uveitis
> - Posterior uveitis
> - Foreign body/corneal abrasion
> - Dry eye
> - Blepharitis
> - Dacryocystitis
> - Dacryoadenitis
> - Orbital cellulitis
> - Periorbital cellulitis

However, topical prophylaxis itself may cause a minor conjunctivitis due to chemical irritation.

Allergic conjunctivitis typically occurs in a child with seasonal allergies and causes eye redness, watering, or itching of the eye. Given the association with seasonal allergies, this conjunctivitis is usually seasonal with pollen exposure or some other allergen. Treatment consists of avoiding the allergen when possible and antihistamines or artificial tears may offer some relief, in addition to antihistamine or mast cell stabilizer eye drop medications.

Although we will not go into great detail, Table 13-1 lists the potential causes of a red eye, which vary from conditions limited to the eye to more systemic diseases, such as autoimmune problems (juvenile idiopathic arthritis, lupus, or inflammatory bowel disease). Most red eyes in children are not going to cause problems, but a few do require urgent evaluation by an ophthalmologist. Some signs to keep in mind that raise concern are decreased vision in the eye, foreign body sensation (like something is stuck in the eye), significant photophobia/sensitivity to light, or trauma to the eye. The presence of one of these signs may mean a more urgent evaluation or referral to an ophthalmologist is needed.

MOVED TO TEARS

Some days it seems that there is not a dry eye in the house...or the pediatric clinic. Eye drainage can come in a variety of forms, from clear tears to goopy, green discharge. Many times, eye drainage accompanies a red eye in conjunctivitis, but occasionally tearing can occur on its own. In young infants, the most common cause of eye drainage or tearing is blocked tear ducts, or congenital nasolacrimal duct obstruction (dacryostenosis). This is caused by an inadequate opening of the tear duct (complete or partial), leaving no opening for the tears to flow so they flow away from the eye and down the face. Occasionally, the eye can be matted shut or have more mucoid drainage. Treatment consists of gently wiping the eyes with warm water and massaging the area over the nasolacrimal duct (between the inner corner of eye and nose). Almost all cases resolve by age 1 year, although a child with prolonged problems may need additional treatment. Infants with nasolacrimal duct obstruction may also develop an infection of this area, called *dacryocystitis*, requiring antibiotic treatment.

Fun Fact: Newborns do not make tears until close to age 1 month.

ENJOY THE VIEW

It is important to watch out for those eyes in children and make sure they see straight, so children can go on playing and exploring and parents can maintain the eyes on the back of their heads.

Chapter 14

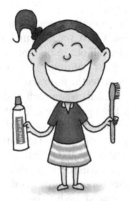

Say Cheese!
(Oral Health)

DEVELOPMENT OF TEETH

Teeth seem like simple little hard structures, but in reality, they are complex living things with various materials, parts, and associated support structures. The precursors of the formed teeth are developed in the fetus during uterine development. The tooth covering, or enamel, is the hardest structure in the body and wraps over all of the other teeth parts. Underneath the enamel

Steiner MJ, Kimple KS. *The Little Book of Pediatrics: Infants to Teens and Everything in Between* (pp 175-181). © 2016 Taylor & Francis Group.

are dentin, cemetum, and pulp layers, and the tooth itself is supported by the bone of the jaw, the ligaments, and the gingiva or gums.

The first teeth generally erupt late in the first year of life. Humans have a first set of primary, or baby, teeth that erupt and later fall out to be replaced by permanent adult teeth. The most common teeth to erupt first are the two lower front teeth, followed by the upper front teeth. Figure 14-1 details when each of the primary teeth erupt and when they generally fall out. Approximately 1 in 2000 babies will either be born with a tooth or have a tooth formed that erupts within the first month of life.[1] Some of these natal or neonatal teeth are malformed, but others are ready to be used as the first primary teeth— although even babies born with a tooth cannot chew or swallow foods that need teeth to be eaten!

As the primary teeth fall out, they are replaced with permanent teeth that need to last the rest of life. In total, most adults will have 32 teeth: 16 on the top and 16 on the bottom. However, the third molars, or wisdom teeth, occasionally do not erupt and stay under the surface of the gums behind the other teeth.

Fun Facts: It is thought that the third molars were named wisdom teeth because they generally erupt late in the teenage years when people are wiser than they were when the other permanent teeth erupted. Now that we know more about brain development, we know that adolescent brain and thought processes are not fully developed until the mid-20s, but late teenagers are still much wiser than elementary school kids. It is believed that the third molars used to be essential because food was less processed and more coarse so teeth used to wear down, even though human lives were much shorter. The third molar was there to share the work! Now, however, with often processed, prepared food and better oral health care, people generally do not need the third molars and they often do not even erupt.

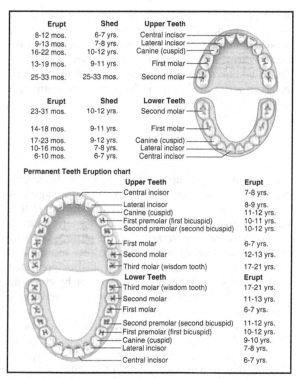

Erupt	Shed	Upper Teeth	
8-12 mos.	6-7 yrs.	Central incisor	
9-13 mos.	7-8 yrs.	Lateral incisor	
16-22 mos.	10-12 yrs.	Canine (cuspid)	
13-19 mos.	9-11 yrs.	First molar	
25-33 mos.	25-33 mos.	Second molar	

Erupt	Shed	Lower Teeth	
23-31 mos.	10-12 yrs.	Second molar	
14-18 mos.	9-11 yrs.	First molar	
17-23 mos.	9-12 yrs.	Canine (cuspid)	
10-16 mos.	7-8 yrs.	Lateral incisor	
6-10 mos.	6-7 yrs.	Central incisor	

Permanent Teeth Eruption chart

Upper Teeth	Erupt
Central incisor	7-8 yrs.
Lateral incisor	8-9 yrs.
Canine (cuspid)	11-12 yrs.
First premolar (first bicuspid)	10-11 yrs.
Second premolar (second bicuspid)	10-12 yrs.
First molar	6-7 yrs.
Second molar	12-13 yrs.
Third molar (wisdom tooth)	17-21 yrs.

Lower Teeth	Erupt
Third molar (wisdom tooth)	17-21 yrs.
Second molar	11-13 yrs.
First molar	6-7 yrs.
Second premolar (second bicuspid)	11-12 yrs.
First premolar (first bicuspid)	10-12 yrs.
Canine (cuspid)	9-10 yrs.
Lateral incisor	7-8 yrs.
Central incisor	6-7 yrs.

Figure 14-1. Primary and permanent teeth with approximate eruption ages.

ORAL HEALTH FOR CHILDREN

Oral health essentially starts immediately after birth, just like the need to take care of other parts of the infant body. Breastfeeding helps support overall infant health and is the perfect food to maintain oral health because breast milk itself does not support the development

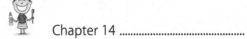
of caries. Speaking of caries, prevention of caries and avoidance of dental trauma are probably the two most important things for early oral health. The habits that are formed early in life around dental care carry on to later life. In addition, the overall oral health of the primary teeth can affect the health of the permanent teeth once they erupt.

CARIES

Caries, or cavities, are acquired defects in the enamel that occur when bacteria in the mouth use sugars as food and create an acidic, damaging environment that starts to literally eat into the tooth. Bacteria hide in plaque and tartar, and scraping off the tartar is one part of the professional cleanings that dentists recommend every 6 months. Caries can be controlled or prevented by decreasing or changing the bacteria or by changing the sugary food environment the bacteria need to do the damage.

Bacteria are present in everyone's mouth. As gross as that is to think about, many of the bacteria are harmless while others can cause cavities. The one type of bacteria that is particularly associated with cavities is called *Streptococcus mutans*. Infants are born with sterile mouths (and generally totally sterile bodies) without bacteria and then slowly acquire bacteria from their environment. We now know that this is one of the ways that severe cavities can "run in families" because bad bacteria can be passed from fathers but especially from mothers to infants. Of course, food in the home and brushing habits are passed down too and affect the rate of cavities, but we know that mothers who partially chew food for infants or put the baby's pacifier into their mouths then they hand it back to the infant increase the risk for early bad bacteria to be present in the baby's mouth and increase the timing and severity of future cavities.

Brushing of the teeth should start upon eruption of the first tooth. Some people even feel that wiping off the gums before the unpleasant eruption of the first tooth can help children get used to oral health care. Some parents use a washcloth or a small brush to do this. There are also small cloths that can fit over the finger for this task. We generally recommend using a tiny bit of fluoride toothpaste to wash those early teeth—and we mean tiny. The amount of toothpaste should be the size of an uncooked grain of rice until age 3 years, when a pea-sized amount can be used. Teeth should be brushed at least twice per day, but ideally they should be brushed (or the mouth should be rinsed out) after each time the child eats food with any sort of sugar in it—which is most food. Drinks containing sugar are particularly bad for the teeth because children often carry around sippy cups that they take sips from over time, so they are constantly exposed to sugar. Those drinks continuously bathe the teeth and the sugar is there for the bacteria to eat. For this reason, children should ideally only drink water between meals and before bedtime.

The introduction of fluoride into the water in the United States has been dubbed one of the Top 10 public health breakthroughs in the history of the country. This has been a big factor in allowing permanent teeth to last as our life expectancy has increased. Although the 70 and 80 year olds of two or three decades ago rarely had their own teeth and usually had at least partial dentures, the future octogenarians who have their own teeth will become the norm. Children who do not drink from public fluoridated water supplies should have their home wells checked for the fluoride level. If the level is low, strong consideration should be given to using a multivitamin with supplemental fluoride. Other than the water supply and fluoride containing toothpaste, there are now fluoride varnishes that can be intermittently painted onto the teeth by health care providers. This is particularly effective for children who are at a high risk for severe cavities. Fluoride prevents cavities by decreasing the ability of the cavity-causing bacteria to create acid and it prevents demineralization of the teeth from bacteria acid. The only known downside to fluoride is that over-dosing on fluoride when the permanent teeth are forming can cause superficial changes in the permanent teeth. Minor changes are mostly cosmetic, but more severe changes can negatively affect the health of the permanent teeth. This will not happen from using publically available fluoridated water supplies or getting small amounts from fluoride toothpaste as described. However, even two to three times this amount of fluoride exposure can cause these changes, so care must be used, like with any ingested substance.

THE OTHER TOOTH FAIRY: DEALING WITH DENTAL TRAUMA

When primary teeth fall out after becoming loose over a period of time, there is obviously nothing wrong with that and it is the expected normal process. However, when trauma or something dramatic causes either primary or permanent teeth to fall out, the child should be evaluated by a dentist.

If a tooth is avulsed or knocked out, there are some steps that families can take to increase the chances that it can be reimplanted. Primary teeth that are knocked out should be saved and taken to the dentist. Avulsion of a permanent tooth is an urgent issue that should be addressed right away. When the tooth comes out, saline solution (like what is used for contact lenses), saliva, or milk can be used to rinse the tooth off. If the tooth fits back into the space and the child is old enough, not trau-matized, and can participate, the tooth can be pushed back into its usual spot while on the way to the dentist. If the child cannot participate, the tooth should be placed in warm milk, saline, or saliva. The tooth should not be put in regular water.

The dentist will examine the other teeth and jaw to make sure there are no other injuries. Everyone knows that sometimes teeth are knocked out; however, teeth can also be injured by being twisted, pushed in, or bent in an abnormal direction. If a tooth was jammed into the gums, the dentist may get an x-ray to determine whether it has harmed the developing teeth or jaw bone beneath it.

Fractured or chipped teeth also need dental evalua-tion within 1 day. Teeth that are deeply chipped can be extremely painful, but even minor chips are places that will easily become infected and develop cavities so den-tists can cover or fill those areas. A lot of dental trauma occurs during activities and widespread use of mouth guards during organized sport and play can dramatically reduce the risk of minor and major injuries to teeth.

REFERENCE

1. Kana A, Markou L, Arhakis A, Kotsanos N. Natal and neo-natal teeth: a systematic review of prevalence and manage-ment. *Eur J Paediatr Dent.* 2013;14(1):27-32.

Chapter 15

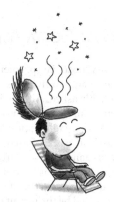

Mind Opener (Psychosocial Health)

The mind is a powerful thing and can even affect the physical health of a child. Concerns about a child's behavior, mental or emotional state, and social well-being are sometimes more common than physical complaints, so providers spend a lot of time addressing these concerns. In addition, psychological problems in children may not be as obvious if providers or parents do not suspect a

Steiner MJ, Kimple KS. *The Little Book of Pediatrics: Infants to Teens and Everything in Between* (pp 183-195).
© 2016 Taylor & Francis Group.

problem, especially because children may present differently or with more somatic complaints than adults.

YOU JUST GOTTA ASK...

Screening for psychosocial problems is especially important because many individuals do not express concern unless explicitly asked. Although discussing psychological well-being can be time consuming, screening tools that are used at well-child appointments make this daunting task a little bit easier. Based on these results, the discussion can be tailored to a particular child. The Pediatric Symptom Checklist is a commonly used tool that consists of 35 questions that relate to emotions and behaviors and is answered by the parent or child (depending on the child's age). Adolescents have a long questionnaire, called the Guidelines for Adolescent Prevention Survey (GAPS), which they fill out at well-child visits. The GAPS form addresses sensitive issues and at-risk behaviors, such as alcohol or drug use, sexual activity, and violence or risk for injuries. Bright Futures also has adolescent health social screening questionnaires. There is a lot to go over during those teenage years, so this form can help providers know where to concentrate and facilitate the conversation. Adolescents should also be routinely screened for depression, and many providers use the Patient Health Questionnaire, which contains nine questions related to depression.

LET'S TAKE A TIME-OUT

Children are not little angels all of the time. Behavioral problems are common and occasionally can be a reflection of an underlying disorder, such as attention deficit hyperactivity disorder (ADHD) or a mood disorder. In addition, many other influences can lead to behavioral problems in children, such as family stressors or divorce, sleep problems, domestic violence, poverty, and foster care. Prior to addressing the behaviors, it is important to understand the behavior and inquire about the child's environment, recent changes, or any other factors contributing to behavioral changes.

INATTENTION IS THE CENTER OF ATTENTION

Problems with attention are becoming more common in childhood and adolescence. Attention deficit disorder or ADHD presents with trouble paying attention, impulsivity, and/or hyperactivity that interferes with functioning both at home and at school. It is important to keep in mind that these symptoms are excessive compared to what is expected at the child's developmental age; for example, a kindergartner may only be able to concentrate for 5 to 15 minutes at a time, but this is normal for his or her age. Not all children with attention problems are jumping off the walls; for example, children with ADHD inattentive type may have trouble in school but may not be disruptive or readily recognized as having a problem paying attention.

Some parents or teachers may raise concerns about a child's attention if issues come up during conversations about school performance. A child may have difficulty sitting still, be fidgety, have trouble listening or following instructions, be easily distracted, daydream, act impulsively or make careless mistakes, and interrupt frequently or be forgetful. These actions must cause a problem in multiple settings, such as in school and at home, and should appear prior to age 12 years to be diagnosed with

ADHD. To make a more objective evaluation of a child's attention and behavior, rating scales can be helpful. The Vanderbilt Rating Scale is a commonly used and valuable tool that is filled out by both the parent and the teacher. This scale looks at problems of inattention and hyperactivity, as well as other behaviors that are suspicious for conduct problems, anxiety, or depression. Anxiety especially is more common among children with ADHD.

It is important to exclude other problems that cause inattention or behavioral issues and look for problems that commonly occur with ADHD. Some children appear to have attention problems or their attention is worse due to other problems, such as learning disabilities, a language disorder, or sleep disorders. If a child has significant trouble in one particular area (eg, reading) or is not improving as expected with treatment, a psychoeducational evaluation can be beneficial to rule out a learning disorder. Learning disorders can masquerade as attention problems, and many children with ADHD also have an associated learning disorder. Trouble with anxiety, depression, family stressors, or lack of sleep can also affect the child's attention and performance in school. Some children with ADHD also have conduct disorder or oppositional defiant disorder. Adolescents with a new onset of symptoms are more likely to have mood disorders, such as depression or anxiety or even substance use. Because ADHD usually has other associated problems, it is important to get the whole picture of what is going on to create the best management approach for the child.

Once a child is diagnosed with one of the three subsets of ADHD (inattentive type, hyperactive/impulsive type, or combined type), treatment consists of medications in addition to possible lifestyle changes, development of coping skills, counseling, and treatment of any comorbid disorders. There are many medications available to treat ADHD, the most common of which are stimulants. Although stimulant medication can help with symptoms of ADHD, it can cause side effects and requires ongoing monitoring by a provider. In addition, these medications have the potential for abuse and some adolescents may use them recreationally.

THE SPECTRUM

Autism spectrum disorder (ASD) is a relatively common neurodevelopmental disorder that is likely present at birth but becomes evident during early childhood, with social interaction and communication problems, as well as repetitive or restrictive behaviors. Some children may also have associated problems, such as intellectual disability, sleep issues, and gastrointestinal issues. The etiology is not completely understood, but most cases may be related to genetic and environmental factors. We do know that vaccines do not cause autism. Previously, there was a distinction between children diagnosed with autism and Asperger disorder, the latter of which are more highly functioning. However, in the most recent fifth edition of the *Diagnostic and Statistical Manual of Mental Disorders*,[1] both are considered ASDs, encompassing a spectrum of varying levels of symptoms and functioning.

The prevalence of ASDs has been increasing, and part of this may be due to increasing diagnosis and alternatively diagnosing autism instead of something else in the past. Most recently, the prevalence is estimated to be about 1 in 68 children and is more common in males than females.[2] Because an earlier diagnosis has been shown to benefit children by getting them into developmental and educational programs, the American Academy of Pediatrics recommends screening at routine well-child appointments.[3] Children are screened with a standardized screening tool specific to autism at the 18- and 24-month well-child visits, in addition to routine assessments of development. A commonly used autism screening tool is the Modified Checklist for Autism in Toddlers. If a provider has concerns about autism or if the child warrants further evaluation based on screening, he or she is referred for diagnosis.

ASD is a clinical diagnosis based on a thorough history, physical examination, and the development and behaviors of the child. The developmental history is particularly important, looking for clues in social and emotional development, speech delay, and abnormal behaviors. ASD can also be a component of genetic disorders, so it is good to get a complete family history and look for signs and symptoms of an underlying genetic problem.

Treatment of ASDs involves a multidisciplinary approach and depends on the child, but has the common goal of improving function and quality of life. Some of the child's deficits can be improved with behavioral and educational therapies while promoting adaptive and coping skills. Some school-aged children may need individualized education plans, whereas others may require placement in a special education classroom. Providers should also treat any comorbid conditions because children with ASD may have other psychiatric problems, such as ADHD, obsessive-compulsive disorder, sleep disorders, or mood disorders.

TEARS AND FEARS

Mood disorders are common in children and adolescents and may not be readily recognized. In addition, a child may have more than one psychological disorder; for example, depression may occur in children with preexisting anxiety, ADHD, oppositional defiant disorder, or even substance abuse. Many kids are reluctant to bring up concerns about mental health, so it is important for providers to ask during visits. Screening in adolescents may bring up concerns that would otherwise not have come up. Asking certain questions may also help kids open up because certain stressors can make a child more vulnerable to depression, such as a family member with depression or mental illness, family problems, violence, recent loss, or struggles with sexual or gender identity. Depression can present with a variety of symptoms, including sad or irritable mood, not finding fun in activities anymore, change in appetite or weight, sleep problems (either trouble sleeping or sleeping all the time), lack of energy, feelings of guilt, problems paying attention or concentrating, and even thoughts of suicide. Young children may have more somatic symptoms, such as headaches or abdominal pain, which may bring them to medical attention. Adolescents can also have varied presentations, from concerning weight loss to worsening school performance. In addition, adolescents may also withdrawal from others, making depression more difficult to recognize by those around them.

Treatment for depression can consist of psychotherapy, medication, or a combination of both. Cognitive behavioral therapy with medication has been shown to be the most effective in treating depression—over either treatment alone. Medications for depression target neurotransmitters in the brain, the most common of which are selective serotonin reuptake inhibitors (SSRIs). These medications can be effective in treating depression but take 2 to 6 weeks to begin working. Although some of these medications are approved for use in children, it is important to discuss the potential side effects and monitor them closely, as with starting any medication. In 2004, The Food and Drug Administration released a black box warning for antidepressants for a possible increase in suicidal thinking or behavior in some children. Although the overall increased risk was small, the risk was higher than in placebo medication. This may be due to the early and incomplete benefits of treatment, such as increased energy, allowing kids to act on previous suicidal thoughts.

Suicide is the third leading cause of death in children aged 10 to 14 years and the second leading cause of death in children aged 15 to 24 years.[4] Therefore, it is critical to take suicidal thoughts, comments, or behaviors seriously. Some children may have to be hospitalized for their own safety, whereas others may be monitored very closely with good support in place. Although the likelihood that a child will act on suicidal thoughts is impossible to determine, there are some factors that increase the risk. Children and adolescents who are actively thinking of suicide, have attempted suicide in the past, are male, have access to a gun, do not have a support system, and have a plan or access to carry out the plan may be more at risk. It is important that those with suicidal ideation have a treatment plan in place in addition to support, close monitoring, observation for warning signs, and information for what to do in an emergency.

Although all kids are going to have anxiety at some point, there are some children who have more pervasive anxiety that causes distress and impaired function. Anxiety disorders are actually the most common psychiatric illness in childhood and, like depression, can co-occur with other psychological conditions. Anxiety disorders include generalized anxiety, social anxiety, panic disorder, specific phobias or fears, or separation anxiety disorder. Other conditions such as obsessive-compulsive disorder, acute stress disorder, or posttraumatic stress disorder are not considered anxiety disorders but do have a component of anxiety.

Anxiety may manifest differently depending on the situation, but symptoms may include difficulty sleeping, changes in eating habits, avoidance, changes in school performance, or somatic symptoms, such as headaches, abdominal pain, or other pain. Children with generalized anxiety will have excessive worries that are difficult to control, such as worrying about school performance, day-to-day activities, or catastrophic events that are often unrealistic. In addition, they may be irritable, restless, or tired all the time and may have difficulty concentrating or trouble sleeping.

Panic disorder is seen more often among adolescents rather than children and relates to a distinct period or time of fear: It is associated with symptoms such as a racing heart beat or palpitations, sweating, trembling, trouble breathing, chest discomfort, nausea, dizziness, or feelings of losing control or doom. These episodes, or panic attacks, can occur due to a particular trigger or for no apparent reason and can lead to the avoidance of certain situations or places. Because these symptoms may also be associated with more serious medical problems, it is important to rule out other medical conditions, such as a heart arrhythmia or hyperthyroidism.

Social or specific phobias can cause intense fear and distress and impair the child's function, rather than a common fear of spiders or just being uneasy in social situations. Most children will have some sort of separation anxiety in the early years or when starting school, but prolonged excessive worry that causes problems can occur. A child may fear that something bad will happen to him or her or to the parent and as a result want to remain with the parent or caregiver at all times, occasionally leading to refusal to go to school.

A good history is key to diagnosing anxiety, and these disorders have certain criteria to make the diagnosis. There are also useful anxiety screening tools that can be used in clinic, such as the Screen for Child Anxiety Related Emotional Disorders or the Multidimensional Anxiety Scale for Children. In addition, the more general Pediatric Symptom Checklist mentioned previously can provide clues to the presence of anxiety. Anxiety disorders can be managed with psychotherapy, such as cognitive behavioral therapy, which provides training for behavioral skills to better cope with anxiety. In addition, medication can be useful in some cases, such as SSRIs.

I WON'T DRINK TO THAT

Depression and other psychiatric illnesses are often associated with an increased risk for substance use and abuse. Substance use can also lead to or worsen mood disorders. Adolescence is a period of adjustment and experimentation, so counseling on the effects, dangers, and negative consequences of substances is beneficial during well-child visits, while reinforcing that most of the conversation can be held in confidence. Alcohol, marijuana, and tobacco are the most common substances used by adolescents, but other drugs and illicit substances are also relatively common. Most adolescents will not become addicts, but substance abuse and addiction are a real risk. In addition, substances are associated with motor vehicle crashes, injuries, and even deaths.

The CRAFFT is a tool used to screen adolescents for risk of substance abuse. CRAFFT is a pneumonic for the questions that relate to being in a Car while under the influence or with someone who was; using alcohol or drugs to Relax; using alcohol or drugs while Alone; Forgetting things while using; Friends or family tell you to cut down; or getting in Trouble while using alcohol or drugs. Substance use has been shown to affect brain development and function, in addition to potential school difficulties, problems with peers, behavior problems or risk-taking, and increased risk of injury. In addition, many youth do not think of substances as being that harmful. Therefore, it is important that providers and the community continue to educate adolescents and try to prevent substance abuse.

Not-so-fun Fact: According to the Centers for Disease Control and Prevention, motor vehicle crashes are the number one cause of death in US teenagers, and for each mile driven, a driver aged 16 to 19 years is 3 times more likely to be in a fatal accident than drivers aged 20 years and older.

SLEEP ON IT

Getting enough sleep is crucial to maintaining good mental and physical health. Some teenagers seek medical attention for feeling tired all the time, which is not surprising after they divulge their sleep habits. Many adolescents are not sleeping enough and have a lot of trouble getting up in the morning, perhaps from the late nights writing a paper, texting, or perusing social media sites. Adolescents are still growing and developing, and sleep is necessary for good brain function. Sleeping until noon on the weekends does not make up for the week's sleep deprivation. Good sleep habits, otherwise known as *sleep hygiene,* are important for everyone, not just adolescents. A consistent sleep schedule with a similar bedtime and wake time each day helps the body return to its natural rhythms. The bed should also be a sleep retreat and not a desk, couch, or kitchen table. Light from the television, computer screens, video games, or cell phone can interfere with good quality sleep, which is an increasing problem because many adolescents have some electronic device in their bedrooms. Caffeine, exercise, or even naps can interfere with sleep if too close to bedtime. Adolescents should be getting at least 8.5 to 9.5 hours of sleep a night, which is hard to do with the need to get up early for school. However, getting good sleep will help with mood, energy, attention, concentration, school performance, learning, and behaviors. So, tell the kids to turn the television and computer off, silence the cell phone, and roll over for a good night's sleep.

MAKING A SCENE OVER THE SCREEN

Children are now reaching for the iPad rather than a book or are sitting in front of the computer instead of playing outside. Given that electronic devices and media constantly surround us, it is important to limit the exposure in children. Excessive screen time has been associated with trouble paying attention, school problems (not all that computer time is "homework"), trouble sleeping, and even obesity. The American Academy of Pediatrics recommends no screen time for children younger than age 2 years because this can interfere with development due to the need to learn from people and the environment...even over Baby Einstein.[5] Older children should be limited to 1 to 2 hours per day, which is a stretch from the average of 7 hours that children are spending in front of a screen.

HAPPY DAYS

Children and adolescents may have minds of their own, but keeping them happy and healthy is an important task. All children should adopt simple behaviors to keep their mind at peace, such as some sort of physical activity each day, eating a healthy diet, getting outside every day, and spending time with family or friends, while also finding some quality time for themselves. Although it can be hard to do in today's busy world, it is amazing what a difference these steps can make.

REFERENCES

1. American Psychiatric Association. *Diagnostic And Statistical Manual Of Mental Disorders, Fifth Edition (DSM-5®)*. Washington, D.C.: American Psychiatric Publishing; 2013.

2. Autism and Developmental Disabilities Monitoring Network Surveillance Year 2010 Principal Investigators. Prevalence of autism spectrum disorder among children aged 8 years – autism developmental disabilities monitoring network, 11 sites, United States, 2010. *MMWR Surveill Summ.* 2014;63(SS02):1-19.

3. Johnson CP, Myers SM. Identification and evaluation of children with autism spectrum disorders. *Pediatrics.* 2007;120(5):1183-1215.

4. Centers for Disease Control and Prevention. National Vital Statistics System, National Center for Health Statistics, CDC. 10 leading causes of death by age group, United States – 2011. http://www.cdc.gov/injury/wisqars/pdf/leading_causes_of_death_by_age_group_2011-a.pdf. Accessed August 6, 2014.

5. American Academy of Pediatrics. Children, adolescents, and the media. *Pediatrics.* 2013;132(5):958-961.

Index

Printed in the United States
by Baker & Taylor Publisher Services